D0146292

*Dealing with Anxiety and
Related Disorders*

Dealing with Anxiety and Related Disorders

Understanding, Coping, and Prevention

Rudy Nydegger

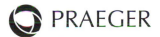 PRAEGER

AN IMPRINT OF ABC-CLIO, LLC
Santa Barbara, California • Denver, Colorado • Oxford, England

Library of Congress Cataloging-in-Publication Data

Nydegger, Rudy V., 1943–
    Dealing with anxiety and related disorders : understanding, coping,
and prevention / Rudy Nydegger.
        p. cm.
    Includes index.
    ISBN 978-0-313-38422-6 (hardback) — ISBN 978-0-313-38423-3 (ebook)
1. Anxiety disorders.   2. Anxiety disorders—Diagnosis.   3. Anxiety
disorders—Treatment.   4. Self-care, Health.   I. Title.
    RC531.N93   2012
    616.85'22—dc23   2011032438

ISBN: 978-0-313-38422-6
EISBN: 978-0-313-38423-3

16   15   14   13   12   1   2   3   4   5

This book is also available on the World Wide Web as an eBook.
Visit www.abc-clio.com for details.

Praeger
An Imprint of ABC-CLIO, LLC

ABC-CLIO, LLC
130 Cremona Drive, P.O. Box 1911
Santa Barbara, California 93116-1911

This book is printed on acid-free paper ∞

Manufactured in the United States of America

This book is dedicated to the memory of my parents, Verne and Jean Nydegger. They always supported and encouraged me and were fun and loving parents. They are missed but with me always.

Contents

Preface   xi
Acknowledgments   xv

1 What Is Anxiety?   1

   The Age of Anxiety   2
   Diagnosing Anxiety Disorders   4
   Diagnostic and Statistical Manual   5
   Multiaxial Diagnoses   6
   Myths about Anxiety   7
   People Who Suffer from Anxiety Disorders   11

2 Living with Anxiety Disorders   15

   Case 1: Betsy   15
   Case 2: Dan   21
   Case 3: Cheri   24

3 The Distribution and Effects of Anxiety Disorders: Costs,
   Gender, Age, and Specific Groups   29

   Gender and Anxiety Disorders   30
      Women and Anxiety   30
      Men and Anxiety   31
   Age and Anxiety   32
      Children and Teens and Anxiety   32
      Diagnosing and Treating Children and Teens   35
      Anxiety Disorders in the Elderly   36
      Treatment of Anxiety in the Elderly   39

Race, Ethnicity, and Anxiety Disorders   39
  African Americans and Anxiety   40
  Asian Americans and Anxiety   42
  Hispanic Americans and Anxiety   44
  Native Americans and Alaskan Natives and Anxiety   45
Homosexual Groups and Anxiety   46
Religious Groups and Anxiety   47

4 Theories of Anxiety Disorders   49
Biological Theories   49
Psychological Theories   54
  Psychodynamic Approaches   54
  Humanistic and Existential Approaches   56
  Behavioral Approaches   58
  Cognitive Approaches   61
Integrating the Different Theories   64
Who Is Vulnerable?   65

5 Physical Responses and Types of Anxiety Disorders I: Generalized
   Anxiety Disorder and Panic Disorder   69
Physical Responses to Stress and Anxiety   69
  Responses of the Brain   69
  Responses by the Heart, Lungs, and Circulatory System   70
  Responses by the Immune System   70
  Responses in the Mouth and Throat   71
  Skin Responses   71
  Metabolic Responses   71
  Physical Responses When Stress or Anxiety
     Disappears or When It Continues   71
  Other Sources of Anxiety-like Symptoms   72
Types of Anxiety Disorders I   73
  Generalized Anxiety Disorder   73
  Panic Disorder   76

6 Types of Anxiety Disorders II: Phobias, Posttraumatic
   Stress Disorder, and Obsessive-Compulsive Disorder   83
Phobias   83
  Specific Phobias   85
  Social Phobia   86
Posttraumatic Stress Disorder and Acute Stress Disorder   89
Obsessive-Compulsive Disorder   99

7   Treatments for Anxiety Disorders   107

    Medical Treatments for Anxiety Disorders   109
        Antidepressant Medications   110
        Antianxiety (Anxiolytic) Medications   111
        Additional Medications and Natural Substances   112
        Pregnancy and Medications   115
        Other Medical Forms of Treatment   116
    Psychological Treatments of Anxiety Disorders   116
    Other Psychosocial Treatment Approaches   119

8   Treatment Methods for Specific Anxiety Disorders
    and Patient Groups   125

    Panic Disorder   125
    Generalized Anxiety Disorder   126
    Social Anxiety Disorder   127
    Specific Phobia   128
    Obsessive-Compulsive Disorder   130
    Posttraumatic Stress Disorder   133
    Other Considerations in Treating Anxiety Disorders   135

9   Living with Anxiety Disorders   139

    Who Needs Treatment?   139
    Where to Seek Treatment   140
    Types of Mental Health Professionals   140
    Is Treatment Working, and When Is It Completed?   145
    What Patients Can Do to Help Themselves:
        Stress Management   147

10 Somatoform Disorders   151

    Malingering and Factitious Disorders   152
    Hypochondriasis   155
    Somatization Disorder   158
    Conversion Disorder   160
    Pain Disorder   163
    Body Dysmorphic Disorder   165
    Other Types of Somatoform Disorders   168

11 Dissociative Disorders   169

    Background and History   169
    Dissociative Disorders in General   171
    Depersonalization Disorder   173

Dissociative Amnesia   173
Dissociative Fugue Disorder   175
Dissociative Trance Disorder   176
Dissociative Identity Disorder   176
Treatments for Dissociative Disorders   180

12   Making Sense of It All   183
Changing Conceptions of Anxiety and Related Disorders   183
Coping with Anxiety and Related Disorders   187
Being a Positive Voice for Good Mental Health   190
Making a Difference   193

Resources   195
References   199
Index   223

Preface

I don't have big anxieties. I wish I did. I would be much more interesting.
—Roy Lichtenstein; American painter, 1923–1997

We live in an age of anxiety is a common phrase for many people that points to a daily life fraught with varying levels of anxiety, stress, trauma, or apprehension. Others may be unaware of the extent to which positive and negative stress can affect our health and daily decisions. In either case, it is not uncommon for people to deny, ignore, distort, or misunderstand symptoms of anxiety, which is only one of the reasons why anxiety and stress-related conditions are frequently untreated.

People who are dealing with worries and difficulties in their lives seldom find lasting comfort from others and may even be offended by comments offered from well-intentioned family members and friends. How often have you been troubled by something only to have someone say to you, "Well, you think that is bad, look at Charlie—his life is falling apart! Your life isn't so bad." Perhaps this was meant to be a source of comfort, but, personally, I have never found comparing someone else's misery to mine an effective way to cheer me up. If it was as easy as, "Just don't think about it!" or "Look on the bright side!" or even, "Don't worry, things will eventually get better!" very few of us would ever experience feelings of anxiety.

Life is filled with people experiencing normal anxieties and stressors, but many live with a higher and prolonged level of anxiety identified as a type of a diagnosable illness called an Anxiety Disorder. This book examines the world of anxiety, including the definition and explanation of its effects, the important differences between normal anxiety and true clinical disorders, and how it is diagnosed and treated. Historically, records from all over the world and for all of our known history show that anxiety and worry have always been an aspect of the human condition. In some communities, people worry from day to day that they will not have enough to eat, a safe place to stay, and the necessities to sustain life. Others worry about their medical condition, relationships, family problems, or world events. One of the differences between anxieties of today and those of yesteryear is the growing number of things we have to worry about, as well as their broadening complexity and pervasiveness. Today's world is more dynamic on many fronts, with the rate of change increasing faster than in previous decades. For example, how many changes in daily living do you think occurred between April 3, 1201, and April 3, 1301, in most parts of the world? How much change has occurred in the lives of people in the developed countries from April 3, 1910, to April 3, 2010? The number of changes that have occurred this year is more than those of last year, and even more will take place next year. The compounded rate of change is itself a major source of stress and anxiety for many. Several decades ago, sociologist Alvin Toffler wrote a book, *Future Shock* (1970), in which the main premise is that people are changing the world faster than they can possibly adapt to the changes, and this reality leads to many social, cultural, and personal problems. It seems clear that many of Toffler's concerns about dealing with life's changes are very true today.

Learning how to recognize and deal with stress, worry, and anxiety is an important challenge for everyone, but for those who struggle with anxiety and related disorders, the difference between managing these disorders and not seeking treatment may be the difference between living a normal, productive, and reasonably happy life and being chronically miserable, uncomfortable, and unproductive. This book examines the issues of living with anxiety, anxiety disorders, and some related psychological problems in a style intended for a broad audience, although professional language and technical terms are used and explained throughout the book as well.

Chapter 1 defines the term *anxiety* and explains how it feels and how it can affect us. Diagnostic issues and controversies related to the detection, diagnosis, and treatment of anxiety and related disorders are discussed, as well as myths and misunderstandings about these conditions. Although everyone has felt anxious or worried at some time, few people understand the real difference between normal worrying and a diagnosable Anxiety Disorder.

Chapter 2 contains three case studies that illustrate the ways in which anxiety disorders have affected the lives of three people. Most people will recognize similarities between patients being treated for Anxiety Disorder and the normal feelings of anxiety that all of us experience, but they will also see some differences between what they experience and the difficulties that these patients face. The case studies were originally drafted by professionals who are experienced with anxiety disorders through education, personal experience, training, and observation. Their effort resulted in a collage of experiences and treatments from different patients but does not reflect any one, single patient. Further, I removed all identifying information from the cases and then rewrote them in a style that is consistent with the rest of the book.

Chapter 3 discusses the demographics and costs associated with Anxiety Disorders, as well as the challenges faced when identifying, diagnosing, and treating different types of individuals. Anxiety Disorders can appear to be similar across cultures or groups, but the differing rates at which anxiety occurs is often unique in some people or communities, and the types of effective treatments can differ as well. Finally, Anxiety Disorders can present differently depending upon sex, age, race, and culture.

Anxiety Disorders can affect people personally, socially, at work, and in school and can impact them in terms of lost work time when going for treatment and appointments, disability, decreased productivity, conflicts at work and in families, lost dreams of success, and damaged or ruined careers and lives. Yet, there seems to be minimal public awareness or concern about the challenges of Anxiety Disorders and how they affect the daily lives of millions of people. Even more troubling is that today there are many different and effective treatments that can minimize and control the misery, expense, and other problems caused by Anxiety Disorders. Unfortunately, treatments are inaccessible in some communities, and some people may not know where to find appropriate treatment or may avoid treatment due to social or cultural stigmas.

Chapter 4 addresses the interesting and controversial issues surrounding the origin and causes of anxiety and similar disorders. Psychological theories range from the psychodynamic, such as Freudian psychoanalysis, to the behavioral approaches and the newer cognitive and cognitive/behavioral approaches, as well as to the humanistic and existential theories. In addition, we will explore some of the sociological and cultural theories and how they impact our understanding of the development and treatment of Anxiety Disorders. How a society or culture views, manages, and pays for the treatment of psychological problems varies widely and is relevant to understanding the causes of Anxiety Disorders. However, these factors alone do not adequately explain the causes, manifestations, types, and treatments of anxiety-related conditions.

Finally, the medical and biological causes, as well as their significant interrelationship with the psychological aspects of anxiety-related problems, are discussed. Some Anxiety Disorders exhibit a strong biological component in terms of apparent causes, symptoms, and treatments, including a possible genetic predisposition in some people.

Chapter 7 examines the most recent research literature on the available and experimental treatments for Anxiety Disorders and explores the advantages and disadvantages of the different types of treatments and the issues involved with their use. Biological, psychological, and alternative treatments are all explored. In Chapter 8, treatment alternatives are explored with special reference to treatments for specific diagnostic categories, and the treatment issues and options for special groups of patients is also addressed. Chapter 9 discusses the issues confronting patients and families of patients with anxiety disorders and goes into more detail about the things that patients and families can do to cope with, help treat, and even prevent some of the problems and complications that are part of having and living with an Anxiety Disorder.

Chapters 10 and 11 discuss two types of disorders that are related to, but not classified as, Anxiety Disorders. Historically, Somatoform Disorders and Dissociative Disorders were considered neuroses and were grouped together with anxiety disorders in the Neurosis category for most of the 20th century. Both Somatoform and Dissociative Disorders involve anxiety and/or trauma to some extent but are now included as separate categories in the *Diagnostic and Statistical Manual of Mental Disorders*, 4th edition (*DSM-IV*), as the term *neurosis* is no longer used.

The last chapter of the book summarizes the issues that have been addressed and discusses some of the treatment, clinical, social, and political issues involved in dealing with these different types of psychological disorders. Finally, appendices at the end of the book list books, articles, organizations, and websites that provide additional resources for people who want or need more information or support as they confront and deal with their anxiety and anxiety-related disorders.

Acknowledgments

No project as large as a book is the result of the work of one person. I would especially like to thank my wife, Karen, who is a fastidious and dedicated proofreader and copyeditor. There is no question that this book is much better for her help and attention. She kept me focused and always had good and important suggestions that clarified and strengthened the material. Her efforts on the book and in providing the support that made it possible for me to take the time necessary to complete this work were amazing, and I truly appreciate and value her contributions to the book and to our family.

Others in my family have always been an enormous source of support as well, and particularly my wonderful, talented, fun, and beautiful kids. My daughters Ashley, Morgen, Colby, and Liesl and my son Austin are a daily source of pride and enjoyment. My grandsons Lucas and Sammy have brought more joy and smiles to my life than I ever would have dreamed. Also, I sincerely appreciate my sons-in-law for their friendship and for being the partners I always hoped my children would find—Jason, Shawn, and Omar, thanks for your friendship and for being the family members that make me proud and grateful.

Finally, I would like to thank my editor, Debbie Carvalko, for her consistent help, guidance, and support. This is my third project with her, and I cannot imagine a better person with whom to work.

1

What Is Anxiety?

Every faculty and virtue I possess can be used as an instrument with which to worry myself.

—Mark Rutherford, British writer, 1831–1913

Anxiety is the one state no one wants to visit. It can take the best of times and make it a terrifying blur of the worst feelings imaginable. It makes you want—no, need to find comfort from anything or anyone, and that is always the wrong thing to do. Anxiety is truly one of the demons of existence.

As awful as this description of anxiety sounds, everyone has felt anxious at one time or another, and it is hardly a unique experience. References to anxiety and fear are found historically in all cultures, and evidence suggests they exist across species. The fight-or-flight reaction is an evolutionary adaptation that helps to protect an organism from harm and mobilizes the body for a quick response. When we feel frightened or anxious, our body readies itself to take action—to resist/fight a threat or to escape/flee from it. However, many people experience intense feelings of anxiety that emerge even when no actual danger is present, yet the body and mind still react as if truly threatened.

Anxiety is a result of the *perception* of threat or danger and is open to wide misinterpretation or distortion. In most cases, anxiety is a future-oriented problem, worrying about something that might happen or exaggerating the perceived threat. When the intensity and duration of the fear is disproportionate to the perceived threat, anxiety is considered maladaptive and unhealthy. Feeling nervous about an upcoming event is certainly normal, but if the anxiety becomes so severe that it prevents us from following through as planned, then the anxiety has developed into a significant problem.

The word *anxiety* is rooted in the Latin word *angere*, which means to choke or strangle.[1] If you have ever experienced acute anxiety, you may remember the feeling of choking or not being able to breathe properly. My own definition of anxiety is "a state of arousal that is subjectively experienced as aversive." In addition, anxiety usually includes feelings of apprehension, uncertainty, fear, and negative thinking. When we are excited about something, our physical reactions are similar to those experienced when we are anxious, but we interpret them very differently. Whether we identify the feelings we experience as anxiety or excitement depends upon the events leading up to those feelings as well as the subjective interpretation of the event or situation.

Symptoms of anxiety include irritability, intense fear, worry, difficulty concentrating, and a general keyed-up feeling. Physical symptoms of anxiety often include sweating, dry mouth, hot flashes or chills, dizziness, heart palpitations, muscle tension, trembling, nausea, and restlessness.[2] When anxiety is very severe, lasts for a long time or frequently recurs, and is disruptive to a person's life and comfort, it may be a diagnosable Anxiety Disorder. Understandably, people who suffer from Anxiety Disorders want desperately to make these feelings and symptoms disappear. One of the best descriptions of severe anxiety is the overwhelming *fear of the loss of control*. This sensation is one of receiving a flood of powerful and crushing negative feelings, a sense that one is dying or that one is losing one's mind that seem completely out of control.

Freud's central theory of anxiety is that it is a signal to us that unwanted and frightening subconscious impulses are trying to gain conscious awareness.[3] Since becoming aware of these thoughts is far too threatening for us to experience consciously, anxiety is, therefore, a warning signal to take action to prevent the thoughts from overwhelming us. Whether anxiety is experienced at the conscious or subconscious level, most theorists and practitioners agree that the fear of the loss of control is central to the experience of anxiety.

THE AGE OF ANXIETY

Many say that we live in an Age of Anxiety, which may seem a bit peculiar considering the numerous comforts and conveniences available to many of us living in a developed country. Why, then, do people who live in relative comfort still experience anxiety to a degree that incapacitates them? The answer is that some people suffer from an Anxiety Disorder, which is the result of a disproportionate response to a *perceived threat* rather than a rational appraisal and response to a *real threat*. Living with an Anxiety Disorder is not the same thing as experiencing normal feelings of anxiety. Millions of people, for whom the perceived threat of harm, illness, and even death is a constant companion, may daily experience a significantly high, and realistic, level of anxiety and fear that is incomprehensible to most of us.

Research indicates that Americans have shifted toward higher levels of anxiety in recent decades, with people in all age groups reporting clinically relevant anxiety more often than ever before.[4] Although this may be due to an increased awareness about mental health issues and more frequently reporting problems, studies show that both children and college students experienced a substantial increase in anxiety between 1952 and 1993,[4] with no indication that this trend has or will subside. During the 1980s, the average American child reported more anxiety than child psychiatric patients of the 1950s, leading some professionals to think that a decrease in social connectedness during our modern times may be responsible for increases in reported anxiety; others think that the world is more dangerous and that increased anxiety is understandable.[4] Certainly, over the past few decades, economic uncertainty, safety concerns, social acceptance, and job security were and are sources of stress, but none of these is a major factor in the rise of diagnosed Anxiety Disorders. The increasing rate of reported Anxiety Disorders in recent years appears to have affected men and women equally, although women still suffer Anxiety Disorders more than men and at about the same rate as in the past.[4] Many authors agree that the 20th century should be referred to as the Age of Anxiety; it remains to be determined if the 21st century will follow suit.

One major difficulty in dealing with anxiety is the manner in which people attempt to control it. I often tell patients who suffer from an Anxiety Disorder that "anything you are presently doing to make yourself feel better is probably the wrong thing to do." That may sound strange, but when we rush to take action without thinking, we often worsen a situation. Likewise, when people notice that feelings of anxiety are beginning to overwhelm them, they want to stop them as quickly as possible. Unfortunately, whatever they typically do will only briefly and temporarily alleviate the anxiety. Some may resort to drugs and/or alcohol in order to self-medicate the anxiety away—but it only works temporarily and often makes the anxiety worse. Others may focus their attention on television, the computer, video games, texting, talking on the telephone, and shopping to distract them from the anxiety, and others may find refuge in food, smoking, or sex. In an effort to control the anxiety, some may display an artificial air of calmness and simply deny that a problem exists. This may at first appear to be someone who is coping, but in reality it is often only denial. An additional misleading coping strategy that can develop into a serious issue is the intentional changing of one's plans or daily routine in order to avoid situations that might produce feelings of anxiety. However, the true source of the anxiety is not the planned event but rather the person's underlying and unrealistic fears in anticipation of the situation. Once you have felt better by having avoided one event, you will go on to avoid a second and third event where feelings of anxiety will surface, and now you have more than two situations that you will need to avoid in order to avoid feeling uncomfortable. The pattern continues until you only have a few places where you can go and feel comfortable. A colleague of mine who lives with an Anxiety Disorder could manage to teach in a classroom, but beyond that he was only comfortable when he was in his office, home, or car. Even when he went to a restaurant, he had to sit by a window to keep his car within view. Fortunately, he sought treatment and went on to live a happy and full life.

DIAGNOSING ANXIETY DISORDERS

In addition to being upsetting and intrusive to one's life, Anxiety Disorders are challenging to diagnose. The professional must determine whether an Anxiety Disorder is present and whether it is a primary or a secondary type of problem or if it is indicative of a totally different disorder. First, it is necessary to determine whether the varying levels of anxiety and fear that people experience are a normal reaction or if they reach the threshold of a diagnosable condition. Research clearly demonstrates that anxiety can be reliably and validly assessed,[5] but that does not mean that it is a simple process; the diagnosis primarily relies upon the clinical judgment of well-trained professionals.

The next challenge when evaluating the symptoms of an Anxiety Disorder is to rule out alternative diagnoses. Because many symptoms of anxiety are physical, the diagnosing professional must consider and ultimately rule out any physical diagnoses as well as alternative psychological diagnoses, and often the collaboration of professionals from different disciplines is helpful or necessary to make a valid diagnosis. When people are acutely anxious, their heart may pound and they may feel as though they are having trouble breathing, both possible signs of a serious medical issue. A medical doctor may suspect that a patient's symptoms are due to anxiety but will run some tests in order to rule out medical problems. For example, someone who is very anxious may report a headache, hot and cold flashes, and nausea—is it anxiety or a virus or some other infection? In addition to physical signs and symptoms, anxiety may accompany other psychological problems, and the diagnostician must be certain that the presenting symptoms of anxiety cannot be better explained by a different diagnosis.

Finally, the professional must evaluate the severity and unique features of the symptoms to determine whether there is a possibility of an illness in addition to the anxiety problem. Other medical or psychological illnesses that are present at the same time as the primary diagnosed condition are known as comorbid conditions. Comorbid conditions can complicate the process of assessing, diagnosing, and treating patients with Anxiety Disorder. However, it is critical that professionals establish a clear diagnostic picture in order to correctly treat any and all of the presenting and relevant conditions.

Although anxiety is an uncomfortable and sometimes frightening condition, it often goes without benefit of a diagnosis or adequate treatment. Those who choose to seek help usually begin with a visit to their primary care physician (PCP), who will first try to rule out physical causes for the symptoms. The PCP may tell the patient that it is nothing serious or to wait and see if the symptoms dissipate on their own, especially if the anxiety is a purely transient problem due to an unusual situation. Second, the PCP might prescribe a psychotropic medication (for psychiatric symptoms) that should ease the burden of the symptoms—a reasonable strategy, particularly on a short-term basis. However, medication alone is rarely adequate treatment for an Anxiety Disorder. Finally, the PCP can refer the patient to a psychologist, psychiatrist, or other appropriate mental health professional for further medication consultation, psychotherapy, or both.

DIAGNOSTIC AND STATISTICAL MANUAL

The *Diagnostic and Statistical Manual*, published by the American Psychiatric Association, is the ultimate source for diagnosing mental disorders and is used by clinicians, researchers, institutions, governmental agencies, and insurance companies to identify and communicate information about patients, to collect statistics, and for insurance billing purposes. Only those who have received specialized training and experience are qualified to use this diagnostic manual. Currently, professionals use the most recent edition, the *DSM-IV-TR* (*Diagnostic and Statistical Manual, 4th Edition, Text Revision*), more often and simply called the *DSM-IV*. It is divided into three parts: the diagnostic category, a set of diagnostic criteria, and a description of each disorder. A specific diagnosis is assigned a three- to five-digit number that identifies its main and subcategory.

The first version of this manual was the *DSM-I* published in 1952, although early efforts to develop a diagnostic system were also attempted by the military and the World Health Organization. In 1968 the revised *DSM-II* was released but was considered to be very rudimentary and still strongly influenced by the psychodynamic point of view, making its applicability somewhat limited. The *DSM-III* was published in 1980 and included a more objective list of diagnostic criteria, followed seven years later by the revised *DSM-III-R*, which was more consistent with the research and theories of the time.

Finally, in 1994 the *DSM-IV* was introduced and included a more systematic and descriptive list of criteria rather than relying on the more interpretive and subjective criteria used in the past. In 2000 the *DSM-IV-TR* addressed some of the complications and weaknesses of the *DSM-IV* and is the current volume used today. Improvements continue on a future *DSM-V*, when new criteria and new categories will be introduced, reflecting the most recent research and theories.

Presently, the diagnoses that are grouped under the heading of Anxiety Disorders in the *DSM-IV-TR* include Panic Disorder (with or without agoraphobia); Agoraphobia without a History of Panic Disorder, Specific Phobia (Simple Phobia); Social Phobia (Social Anxiety Disorder); Obsessive-Compulsive Disorder; Posttraumatic Stress Disorder; Acute Stress Disorder; Generalized Anxiety Disorder (Includes Overanxious Disorder of Childhood); Anxiety Disorder Due to a General Medical Condition; Substance-Induced Anxiety Disorder; and Anxiety Disorder Not Otherwise Specified. All of these conditions will be explored in this book, and we will examine some of the symptoms, causes, and treatments for each disorder.

MULTIAXIAL DIAGNOSES

Following a thorough assessment according to *DSM-IV-TR* criteria, the patient is assigned diagnoses, which are divided into five parts: Axes I, II, III, IV, and V. The multiaxial system provides different information on the functioning levels of a patient, ranging from a specific and immediate psychological illness needing treatment to other medical, social, and environmental conditions that impair and impact a patient's life. The disorders discussed in this book are primarily Axis I, but some conditions (e.g., Personality Disorders) are included from the Axis II category. The following multiaxial diagnoses are currently used:

Axis I: Clinical Disorders, and
  • Other Conditions That May Be a Focus of Clinical Attention
Axis II: Personality Disorders, and
  • Mental Retardation
Axis III: General Medical Conditions
Axis IV: Psychosocial and Environmental Problems
Axis V: Global Assessment of Functioning

Treating a patient includes a comprehensive diagnosis on all five axes, although the Axis I diagnosis is typically the main focus of treatment. When discussing a course of treatment for an Anxiety Disorder patient, *all* comorbid conditions, including Axis II and Axis III conditions, must be carefully considered as well as the impact of any Axis IV issues. Axis V is often used as an indicator of functional impairment and can be used as a benchmark for assessing treatment progress.

MYTHS ABOUT ANXIETY

Understanding the nature and impact of Anxiety Disorders means separating the many myths and misconceptions from the facts. Popular thinking and discussions on these issues are rarely based on modern theories and research and are not usually consistent with standard diagnostic criteria. Therefore, we will address some of the myths and the facts that will hopefully clarify them.

Myth: Anxiety Conditions Are Rare

Fact: Although most people do not suffer from a diagnosable Anxiety Disorder, these types of disorders are not rare. About 19 million Americans suffer from a clinically relevant Anxiety Disorder, and it is likely that you know someone who lives with severe anxiety.[1] A list of well-known people who have publicly acknowledged dealing with Anxiety Disorder is presented at the end of this chapter.

Myth: Anxiety Disorders Are Not Illnesses

Fact: Although Anxiety Disorders are not caused by a particular germ or passed around like a cold virus, they are legitimate psychiatric illnesses identified by specific set of symptoms and diagnostic criteria found in the *DSM-IV*. Several psychological as well as physical factors are involved in the development of Anxiety Disorders.

Myth: Only One Type of Anxiety Disorder Exists

Fact: There are several categories and types of Anxiety Disorders, each differing in appearance and symptoms, course and progression, and in the types of treatments required. Although debilitating anxiety is common to all Anxiety Disorders, disorders may appear quite differently in different people, and ways of coping with Anxiety Disorder vary greatly.

Myth: An Anxiety Disorder Is a Fixed Element of Personality

Fact: Although some people are more inclined to feel anxious as part of their personality, an Anxiety Disorder is not a component of one's personality, but rather is acquired *in addition to* the personality. Anyone can develop an Anxiety Disorder, and some may be more prone than others due to genetics, past experiences, or even their personality. But an Anxiety Disorder is not an ingrained, fundamental part of an individual's personality. Treating an Anxiety Disorder means reducing and controlling the symptoms, not changing the patient's personality.

Myth: Emotionally Immature People Develop Anxiety Disorders

Fact: There is absolutely no relationship between emotional maturity and the development of an Anxiety Disorder. The causes of these types of disorders are based entirely on other factors and do not reflect someone's level of maturity, accomplishments, or personal strengths or convictions. Strength lies in seeking treatment, not in denying the need for it. Women are more frequently diagnosed with Anxiety Disorders because they are more willing to receive treatment and are more often affected by complex factors such as genetics and social roles. These will be discussed in depth later in this book.

Myth: Parents Cause Anxiety Disorders

Fact: Developing an Anxiety Disorder involves complex processes and does not arise from a single or simple source. Rarely do all of the children within one family develop Anxiety Disorders, despite the shared environment. Children of conscientious parents can develop Anxiety Disorders, while children of less competent parents can grow up without an Anxiety Disorder and vice versa. All parents can look back and think of things they might have done differently, but their treatment of their children cannot be the *only* factor that produces Anxiety Disorders. However, genetic factors can certainly be a factor to consider when noting frequent occurrences of Anxiety Disorder within one family.

Myth: Medical Conditions Cause Anxiety Attacks

Fact: Although anxiety attacks exhibit physical symptoms—including racing or irregular heartbeat, trouble breathing, and chest pain—they are not the result of a physical problem, such as a heart attack, nor will they make a heart attack occur. Still, many frightened people who are gasping for breath and consumed by thoughts of imminent death rush to a hospital emergency room believing they are having a heart attack. At such times, it is difficult to remember that *no one has ever died as a result of an anxiety attack*. People who have never experienced an anxiety attack cannot even imagine the terrifying and intense feelings and symptoms that are involved.

Myth: Avoiding Stressful Situations Controls Anxiety Attacks

Fact: Avoiding more situations perceived to be responsible for feelings of severe anxiety will not alleviate symptoms but rather exacerbate them. Treatment methods are intended to support a person while confronting difficult or new situations rather than avoiding them. Focusing on efforts to *not* avoid those situations that produce severe anxiety is a major component of psychological treatments for Anxiety Disorders.

Myth: Intense Feelings of Anxiety Mean the Person Is Losing Control

Fact: The most significant word in understanding severe anxiety is the *fear* of losing control, not actually losing control. A person may feel as if she cannot control what is happening to her, but in reality she *does* have control over her own behavior as well as control over her reactions to the fear and/or anxiety she is experiencing. In fact, most treatments for Anxiety Disorders are based upon methods that teach people how to gain control over their actions, thoughts, and feelings within their own unique circumstances in order to reduce and/or eliminate the anxiety.

Myth: You Can Pass Out During an Anxiety Attack

Fact: An anxiety attack does not by itself cause someone to faint. However, if someone is hyperventilating (breathing too fast for too long), he may become light-headed and could briefly lose consciousness, although this is very rare. Even if this were to occur, one would have plenty of time to react (for example, when driving a car, one would have plenty of time to pull the car over to a stop). Refusing to drive a car and isolating at home is a good example of how the *fear* of having an anxiety attack can lead to additional problems. That is why treatment involves helping people learn how to avoid or minimize the intensity of an anxiety attack using psychological techniques.

Myth: Responsible People Often Worry

Fact: Acting responsibly has nothing to do with worrying. However, frequent worrying has a lot to do with being continuously anxious. People who are chronic worriers often spend inordinate amounts of time thinking about things they cannot do anything about. Focusing one's time and actions on those issues that are under your own control is a much more constructive use of one's energy. One step in the treatment for Anxiety Disorders is learning how to avoid unnecessary worrying.

Myth: Worrying May Prevent an Unwanted Event from Occurring

Fact: This is called *superstitious thinking* and is clearly not rational. Most people realize that what they are thinking has nothing to do with when or why things happen. However, some people justify chronic worrying by explaining that it prepares them to deal with a feared, unwanted outcome more effectively than being surprised by it. But being prepared is not equivalent to worrying about an event until it finally occurs. Continuous thinking and worrying about the worst-case scenario is neither realistic nor healthy and is a waste of time and energy. It does not produce the necessary skills or motivation to confront and deal with problems and can lead to needless, dysfunctional symptoms and to avoidance.

Myth: Thinking Positive Thoughts Eliminates Anxiety Disorders

Fact: Depending upon positive thinking as a cure for an Anxiety Disorder is similar to *superstitious thinking* as mentioned above. Trying to control anxiety by thinking "happy thoughts" may temporarily alleviate some feelings of stress, but it is not a cure. Thinking about something does not change the occurrence or outcome of an event. However, some benefits to positive thinking are proving to be important in terms of treatment, theory, and research. Learning to control our actions, thoughts, and feelings is a productive and significant element of most treatment methods, but positive thinking is not a treatment by itself.

Myth: Identifying the Original Cause Fixes an Anxiety Disorder

Fact: Over time an Anxiety Disorder becomes "functionally autonomous," which means that it exists independently of its original cause(s). Behavior patterns that develop help us to practice the anxiety symptoms over a lifetime and need to be addressed, regardless of the precipitating events or remote history behind them. Fragmented and inaccurate memories cannot produce a reliable picture of past personal events, and focusing only upon the suspected source of the Anxiety Disorder is rarely effective or desirable. In addition, the original cause of an Anxiety Disorder may never be discovered.

However, it does serve the entertainment industry well, as is often seen in movies or television shows where the "super shrink" identifies the hidden cause of a person's lifetime of misery, and, through the magical and powerful treatment du jour, the character is miraculously cured and lives happily ever after. If it was only that simple!

Myth: Medications Mask Symptoms and Do Not Cure Anxiety Disorders

Fact: Some people believe that you cannot treat Anxiety Disorders with medication because the drug only covers up the symptom and prevents actual treatment from working. In reality, prescription drugs are not a cure but rather a tool—preferably used in conjunction with psychotherapy—to reduce, control, and eliminate symptoms of severe anxiety. Using medication as the *only* treatment over a long period may result in the return of Anxiety Disorder symptoms once the medication is discontinued. Occasionally, medication alone may be adequate treatment for someone who develops an Anxiety Disorder in reaction to a specific and recent situation, but only on a short-term basis. Recent evidence suggests that, when used improperly, medications can interfere with the effectiveness and long-term benefits of psychotherapy, which is why the psychologist/therapist and prescribing professional must work together.

Myth: Simple and Easy Treatments for Anxiety Are Available

Fact: Anxiety Disorders are complex and their treatments are not simple. When you read or hear, "Get rid of your anxiety in a matter of hours or days—just buy this book, and your problems will be over"—save your money! Quick cures found on the Internet, as well as promises for a new treatment, which psychologists and psychiatrists are somehow unaware of, often dupe unsuspecting people into wasting money and hope on worthless and potentially damaging information. Also, cults and cultlike organizations, claiming to have developed successful treatments for psychological problems such as anxiety, induce desperate people to pay large sums of money in exchange for a cure. It cannot be stressed enough that both the development of and treatment for Anxiety Disorders involves complex processes that cannot be understood or treated with simple-minded and unrealistic methods that were designed primarily to separate people from their money.

Myth: Only Treatment "X" Is Effective on Anxiety Disorders

Fact: No two patients are alike, and the treatment that works for one may not work for another. Experienced professionals know which types of therapies and medications are most likely to work and will develop a treatment plan that carefully considers the full range of possibilities. They must discuss the treatment plan with the patient, including both the benefits and potential risks of treatment options; make a recommendation; and then begin treatment.

Learning the facts rather than the myths about Anxiety Disorders will help you to begin to understand what causes them, how they are treated, and how they affect us. Having accurate information can help someone seek needed treatment; read, talk to your friends who are in treatment, and discuss issues or ask questions of your primary care physician and other professionals.

PEOPLE WHO SUFFER FROM ANXIETY DISORDERS

Everyone knows at least one person who suffers from an Anxiety Disorder, although you might not know it by looking at them. With treatment, most people can live a normal life, whether the anxiety is an acute or chronic problem. Learning how to control and minimize the symptoms is one of the fundamental elements of treatment; being able to effectively deal with situations that produce anxiety is the other.

In addition to negotiating a life without the normal boundaries of privacy, a number of famous and talented people suffer from Anxiety Disorders. Some of these celebrities have been forthcoming about their condition, and their openness has given hope to others who deal with similar disorders. Many historical figures have been written about or have written about their own personal challenges with Anxiety Disorders. The following list of well-known people who suffer from Anxiety Disorders gives you an idea of how widespread and common these problems are:

- Isaac Asimov (author)
- Kim Basinger (actor)
- David Bowie (singer)
- Charlotte Brontë (author)
- Barbara Bush (former first lady of the United States)
- Nicholas Cage (actor)
- Earl Campbell (football player)
- Ray Charles (musician)
- Cher (singer, actor)
- Eric Clapton (musician)
- Michael Crichton (author)
- Sheryl Crow (musician)
- Johnny Depp (actor)
- Emily Dickinson (poet, writer)
- Sally Field (actor)
- Aretha Franklin (singer)
- Sigmund Freud (psychoanalyst)
- James Garner (actor)
- Goldie Hawn (actor)
- Anthony Hopkins (actor)
- Michael Jackson (singer, entertainer)

- Naomi Judd (singer)
- Nicole Kidman (actor)
- Courtney Love (singer, actor)
- John Madden (former NFL coach, sports announcer)
- Howie Mandel (comedian, TV host)
- Alanis Morissette (singer)
- Donny Osmond (singer, actor)
- Marie Osmond (singer, entertainer)
- Bonnie Raitt (musician)
- Burt Reynolds (actor)
- Joan Rivers (comedian)
- Carly Simon (singer)
- John Steinbeck (author)
- Howard Stern (radio personality)
- Barbra Streisand (singer, actor)
- Ricky Williams (professional football player)
- Oprah Winfrey (media mogul)

A specific type of Anxiety Disorder called Obsessive-Compulsive Disorder (OCD) will be explained in chapter 6. Some celebrities who suffer from OCD include:

- Woody Allen (actor, director)
- Dan Aykroyd (actor)
- Alec Baldwin (actor)
- Roseanne Barr (comedian)
- David Beckham (professional soccer player)
- Ludwig van Beethoven (composer)
- Penelope Cruz (actor)
- Charles Darwin (scientist, author)
- Cameron Diaz (actor)
- Leonardo DiCaprio (actor)
- Fred Durst (musician)
- Albert Einstein (physicist)
- Harrison Ford (actor)
- Kathie Lee Gifford (TV host)
- Jennifer Love Hewitt (actor)
- Michelangelo (artist, engineer)
- Martin Scorsese (director, producer)
- Billy Bob Thornton (actor)
- Justin Timberlake (singer, entertainer)
- Donald Trump (businessperson, entrepreneur)[6]

It is encouraging to see how many accomplished people have successfully dealt with anxiety in their lives. Some types of Anxiety Disorders are more chronic than others, but it is possible to receive treatment that will help to manage and even cure the problem. A chronic psychological condition requires continuous monitoring, as does a chronic medical condition such as diabetes—if you take care of yourself and are compliant with treatment you can live a normal and fulfilling life.

2

Living with Anxiety Disorders

Worry is a thin stream of fear trickling through the mind. If encouraged, it cuts a channel into which all other thoughts are drained.
—Arthur Somers Roche, American writer
and screenwriter, 1883–1935

The following three case studies describe the personal experiences of three people who live with Anxiety Disorder. Each of the case studies was originally drafted by professionals who, through education, personal experience, training, and observation, are experienced with Anxiety Disorders. Their efforts resulted in a collage of events and treatments, but each case study does not reflect any one, single patient. All identifying information was removed from each case, and the cases were rewritten in a style consistent with the rest of the book.

CASE 1: BETSY, 26-YEAR-OLD SINGLE WOMAN, NEVER MARRIED, NO CHILDREN

From my first memories as a child, I never felt normal and always knew that I was somehow different from the other kids. It seems as if I was always scared or worried about something. It never seemed like I was having as much fun as the other kids. The things that most kids laughed and teased each other about were things that often upset me or ruined my day. For example, when I was in the second or third grade, we were sitting in a circle during our reading group, and I was sitting next to a girl I didn't know very well, but she made some kind of noise. I looked over at her, then down at her book in her lap to see what she was reading. I immediately noticed something on the book—it was some kind of mess. It looked like she had thrown up on the book, and I panicked. I was very nervous and felt like I was going to be sick— I was frightened to death. My heart was pounding. I started sweating, and I felt like I had to run out of there as fast as I could.

When the little girl saw that I was upset, she said to me, "I'm sorry—I just sneezed, that's all." She looked at me like I was weird or something! Whatever *it* was seemed so disgusting to me and really grossed me out. I immediately asked to go to the bathroom, and the teacher gave me a pass (I knew she could see that something was wrong). I walked as quickly as I could to the bathroom (remember, no running in the halls). Immediately I went to the sink and washed my hands—over and over again. I must have washed my hands 30 or 40 times; each time I had to pump the soap three times.

I returned to the classroom and found that everyone had already returned to their seats, but my book was still lying there on the floor. Although the other girl hadn't sneezed on *my* book, I felt as if mine was contaminated, and there was simply no way I was going to pick up the book. So I just left it there and took my seat. The teacher noticed the book still lying on the floor, picked it up, and put it on my desk, but I still wouldn't touch it. She asked me if I needed to go to the nurse, but at this point I was so embarrassed I just wanted to disappear. So, I said no. From that moment on, it was though *all* of the books at school were now contaminated. When I had to touch one, I would grit my teeth and do it, but then I had to go straight to the bathroom at the first opportunity and thoroughly wash my hands; although, in all honesty, my hands never felt clean. I never finished reading that book; I didn't turn in my book report; and I took a zero on the assignment. The zero was very tough for me to accept, because I have always felt that I needed to receive the best grade in the class. From that time forward, school was awful for me. I felt dirty and contaminated all of the time. Instead of having fun with my friends and learning new things, I always worried about germs and diseases and couldn't wait to get home to take a shower (I can't take baths—sitting in filth that washes off of your body is way too much for me).

This is one of the most dramatic events in my memory, but I know I had issues with being uncomfortable even before that. I can't remember ever not being anxious. As a toddler I kind of remember always hiding behind my parents' legs when strangers came up to us. I have seen photos, and others have told me that I was the most shy child they had ever seen. I wasn't shy; I was terrified! When I was invited over to someone's house to play or to sleep over, I always had a reason why I couldn't go and usually asked my parents to lie for me so I didn't have to go. I knew there was no way that I could tolerate being away from my "safe place" and be around the dirt, germs, and nastiness I knew that I would find in others' homes. Of course, our house wasn't perfect, but my parents thought it was cute and precocious that I was so neat and clean and would often brag about me to their friends. When I heard other parents say, "I wish my kids were more like your daughter," I knew they were unaware of how frightened and miserable I was.

At about age seven my folks insisted that I sleep over at my best friend's house, and, as frightened as I was, I did it. As an only child I always clung tightly to my parents, and they simply wanted some time to themselves. I tried—I really, really did, but it was just too much for me. At 2:00 A.M., my friend's mother called my folks saying that she could not get me out of the bathroom; I couldn't stop washing my hands and crying. That was the last time my parents ever made me do that. So, when did the anxiety start? I think that I was probably anxious in the womb.

I often wonder why I am so different from others. Even in my own family there is no one like me. Well, maybe that isn't exactly true. Both of my parents are fairly neat and clean, but especially my mom wants everything to be "just so." But she doesn't freak out the way I do. I remember my grandma (mom's mother) coming for a visit—I loved her, and she was wonderful to me. However, before her visits my mother would wash, wax, and clean until everything was perfect. I remember her telling my dad, "Please help me; you know how she is." When grandma finally arrived, I was so excited to see her. She always brought me something special, and we would sit together and read and play games. Then I remembered why her visits seemed to last forever. She constantly corrected my mother, telling her that she wasn't doing something right or that something else was dirty and needed cleaning—mom couldn't do anything right. Grandma came into my room every morning and criticized how I or my mother made my bed. She would take the blanket and sheets off of the bed and remake it—several times, until it was exactly right. She instructed me on the need to learn how to do things properly so I wouldn't turn out to be a slob like my mom. I loved her, and know that my mother did too, but grandma was a bit of a stitch (to use one of her own words).

There is no doubt that my problems created difficulties for me all my life. At home, I know that I was a source of conflict between my parents. Mom felt that I was just sensitive and that they should let me do whatever was comfortable for me. So what if I took long showers, washed my hands a lot, and turned on and off every light switch three times going in and out of each room! Dad thought they were spoiling me, that I was weird and needed to shape up if I was ever going to make it in the world.

My parents liked to travel and take vacations, but if I couldn't get there by car in a few hours or if I had to sleep in a dirty hotel bed, there was no way I was going. They tried to drag me onto a plane going to Disney World, but I made such a scene in the airport that the airline people would not permit my folks to board the plane with me. Mom was devastated, and dad was furious. That seemed to be the beginning of the end for them, and they started to drift apart. We never ate dinner together anymore; in the evenings mom did paperwork, and dad watched TV—I just tried to be invisible and wash up as often as I could sneak into the bathroom. They finally divorced, and my mom and I remained in our house. Dad picked me up sometimes, but I wouldn't stay overnight at his house—way too dirty. After awhile he stopped coming to visit me. As much as I loved and missed him, I was glad I didn't have to go there anymore. Yes, I blame myself for my parents' divorce, and there is nothing anyone can say to me that can make me think otherwise.

My social life at school and with friends—right, like I had friends—was virtually nonexistent. I earned good grades in school, because I didn't do anything but study. I played cello in the orchestra, and I was pretty good, but I could never go on trips to perform. Eventually, I was dropped from the group—fine by me; I didn't want to be around all of those disgustingly dirty people anyway. Most people thought I was weird and stuck up. I rarely talked to anyone, and as a result they thought that I considered myself too good for them. In reality, I thought that I was so screwed up that I couldn't risk letting anyone know that I was such a basket case. I was sorry people didn't like me, but it actually made it easier for me. I didn't have to continually make up excuses why I couldn't go to parties and games, try out for sports or cheerleading (which I really wanted to do), be in a play, or have a boyfriend. There was no way I could have allowed myself to be in any of those situations. Holding it together until I returned home and disinfected myself was about all I could manage.

Following high school graduation, everyone assumed I would go away to college, but I knew it was too much for me to handle. Instead, I took some online courses, earned a certificate in medical transcription, and got a job working from home. This was also about the same time when I began to experience serious problems with my nutrition. While in school, I trusted my mother to pick out and prepare my food at home. When I started to work, mom told me that I needed to be more independent and to look for my own apartment. As scary as that was, and as much cleaning as it would require, I finally did move into a place that was all mine. However, now I had to buy my own groceries, which led to me worry about fat grams, carbs, calories, and all of that stuff. Then, I developed a new worry: gaining weight. I bought some workout CDs, watched my diet, and exercised at home. I noticed that I was losing hair, my weight was way down (which worried my mom), I was lightheaded most of the time, and I usually felt nauseous. I went to the doctor, who read me the riot act. I met with a nutritionist and returned to the doctor weekly for a weight check. Although I started gaining weight and eating healthier, frequent visits to the doctor led to two new problems: worrying about catching some disease and driving the doctor's office nuts—that's funny; I was the nut, but I was making everyone around me nutty. I was quickly on a first-name basis with the office staff and was treated well. They were very reassuring and ultimately saved my life by referring me to the professionals who were able to help me.

Until very recently, my life was really pathetic. My daily routine was: eat breakfast, clean up, work out, and do my typing. The company loved me because I was the fastest and most productive typist in the whole group. They often asked me to come to the office for more training or to meet with my supervisors, but I always gave a good reason why I couldn't make it. However, my work was so good that they never forced the issue. My social life consisted of going to mom's and the grocery store, getting my car serviced, and staying at home. For a short time I had another job in a clothing store. At first I was a real hero. I cleaned the store, straightened the clothes, refolded the shirts and sweaters—all of the stuff that no one else wanted to do. Of course, they didn't realize that I was doing it because I couldn't stand the mess or to have the clothes out of order. However, problems soon began when they promoted me to assistant manager, which included opening the store. As long as I arrived early enough to perform all of my rituals, all went well. The lights had to be turned on and off three times; the door had to be opened and closed three times; I had to close my locker three times—you get the idea. I had to—and I mean *had* to—do each task in threes. Usually, I am very good at disguising my rituals, but having so many different responsibilities when opening the store, it was bound to catch up with me—and it did. My first task when arriving at the store was to disarm the security alarm. Of course, the code could only be put in one time, and it bothered me that I couldn't repeat it twice more. But I just couldn't let it go at that. In order to allow myself two more repetitions on the code, I rationalized that, since I had turned the alarm off the first time, I could now safely turn it on and off very quickly two more times without it making a difference. Of course, after I tried this once, the police showed up and had to turn off the alarm. They called my boss, who was furious—I was fired on the spot.

I also tried to develop a social life. I met a guy at the store one day who seemed nice and asked me out to dinner. I knew I couldn't handle that. I couldn't agree to have drinks, because I am afraid to drink; I might lose control and do something awful—nothing sexual or anything—just getting dirty and not being able to wash or fulfill all of my rituals, the stuff I could never explain to someone. So, we settled for meeting for coffee. He was nice and very pleasant and wanted to see me again, and I agreed to meet him for lunch the following week. However, I was so nervous while getting ready that I ran out of time to do all of my rituals. I wasn't sure that I had completed my shower ritual, so I took three more showers to make sure I got it right. I forgot to do the light switch three times in my room, so after I was dressed I had to undress, go back and take another shower, go into the room the right way, turn on and off the lights three times, and finally get dressed again. By the time I was ready, I was an hour late for lunch. I was so mortified that I decided that I couldn't go at all—I couldn't even talk to him again. When he tried to call me, I just ignored his calls, and he finally stopped calling. I still feel terrible about it, but it proved to me that I can never have a relationship with someone. After all, who could possibly put up with someone as crazy as me?

As you might guess, my mom took me to see many shrinks. I saw psychologists, social workers, psychiatrists, but no one helped much. They diagnosed me with depression and anxiety, and for sure I had both. But since I had done such a good job of covering up my other symptoms and I never told anyone about them, no one diagnosed the true problem. Much later I discovered that I had Obsessive-Compulsive Disorder (OCD). If you ask me, a better name would be Excessive Repulsive Disorder—I am sick of having it ruin my life.

Finally, one day I decided that enough was enough. I went to my mom's house and told her about everything. Of course, she had already figured it out. When I was younger she just thought I would outgrow it, and when I was older she felt so guilty that she didn't know what to say or do—so she didn't do anything. She called around to find a psychiatrist who treated OCD and made an appointment for me. I was scared to death, but I went to see him. He was a nice man who explained OCD and said that I needed to take some medication to begin controlling my symptoms. If I was going to get better, I also had to see a psychologist who could work with me to help rid myself of the repetitive thoughts that had plagued me since childhood—all of the worrying about germs, contamination, illness, and so forth was finally going to be challenged and treated. My psychiatrist recommended a clinical psychologist who worked with OCD patients, and the two doctors became my treatment team and also included my mom and me. I eventually learned how to manage the obsessions and compulsive rituals that have plagued me for most of my life.

I have now been in treatment for about a year and am finally beginning to see some hopeful signs. The OCD is not gone, and, in fact, they tell me that I might be dealing with it for the rest of my life. But I am beginning to believe that *I* can control *it* and not the other way around. I am certainly not where I want to be yet, but I am much better than I was before. I still have my typing job and work part-time job in a different clothing store. I straighten the shelves, but only as needed, and I sell clothes and work the cash register without worrying about catching germs from the keys or customers. I even had a date recently, and guess what? He likes me and wants to take me out again. I really can't believe that I may finally have a real life—I cry when I think about it.

I don't regret the past years or blame my parents. Who knew what OCD was and what to do about it back then? I certainly didn't. I just knew that I was crazy and couldn't let anybody know. Well, now I know that I am not really crazy, but I have a disorder that can be controlled and treated. I even got in touch with my dad after all of these years. We cried and laughed together on the phone, and we can't wait to see each other. He now lives in another city and is driving in to see me. He hopes that someday I will be able to get on a plane and fly out to visit him—or drive if I want to. I am so thankful for my new life that I can hardly wait to get up in the morning to see what the new day will bring. My advice to others who suffer from similar problems? Get help, listen, and do what they tell you to do. Don't let embarrassment keep you from going for treatment. There is no reason to be miserable any longer when there are professionals who can help.

CASE 2: DAN, 38-YEAR-OLD MAN, MARRIED WITH TWO CHILDREN

A few years ago I went out with a few of my friends—a real treat, as I rarely go out socially without my wife. She suffers from fibromyalgia and is exhausted and in pain most of the time and prefers to stay at home. I love her very much and want to be supportive of her, the kids, and the household chores as much as possible. However, this one evening she insisted that I go out for an evening of dinner and bowling with some friends from work. While eating at the restaurant, we discussed our childhoods and where we grew up. Suddenly, I became very nervous but didn't know why. When they asked me questions about growing up, I told them where I had lived but couldn't remember much more. I made up a few things and then changed the subject very quickly. They noticed that I was upset and didn't push the issue, but I could tell they thought that I was acting a little strange.

At home that evening I sat down trying to recall my childhood, but I only remembered fragmentary moments. The more I dwelled on it, the more anxious I became. Finally, I had to get to bed and try to fall asleep and forget—isn't that interesting?—trying to forget about my forgetting! The next morning I awakened even more nervous and decided that I had to discover what was wrong with me. It had never occurred to me before that I didn't remember much of my childhood—it was never an issue before.

My dad died a few years ago of a heart attack. After moving to Florida, my parents didn't like to travel to the cold Northeast, so we didn't see them often. My dad was a stern man who didn't talk much, and when we phoned them mom was usually the one to speak with us. Although I never visited them in Florida, my brother and sister had gone with their families a few times and always said that the visits were never pleasant. In fact, they usually used our folks' house as a place to stay while visiting the theme parks and did the usual Florida touristy stuff. I was never interested in visiting, and with my wife's health it was never a consideration.

I called my mom to ask how she was doing and to ask a few questions about my childhood. She was glad to hear from me and asked about my wife and kids, and talked about the weather, her clubs, and friends, and invited us for a visit. When I again broached the subject of my childhood, she clammed up and didn't say much. She offered a few sparse details but claimed that her memory wasn't what it used to be. I decided that she just didn't want to talk about it. So there I was; no memories of my family before I left for college, and no help from my mother.

Next I called my brother and sister, who shared with me events that I don't remember. In the past they didn't speak about our family's history because I never wanted to. Finally, a story of violence and abuse emerged. Apparently, my dad was a raging, violent man who terrified and terrorized our family. I was the eldest and, therefore, was always the primary target. My siblings would receive spankings but that was about all. No one said that they ever saw him hit my mother, but my brother and sister said that mom was absolutely scared stiff whenever he was home, especially if he was angry—which was most of the time. They also told me that I was the scapegoat, the example, and the main target of his rage and abuse. Everything I did was wrong, and every punishment was a horror. Although I can't remember any of it, I was told that I was regularly beaten, whipped with a belt, humiliated, locked in a closet for hours, frequently forbidden to eat meals, and held up to ridicule for virtually everything I did. My siblings felt awful for me but never said anything to mom or to anyone else about the abuse because they were afraid they would then become dad's newest targets. I recently heard the phrase, "conspiracy of silence"; that was my family.

As one might imagine, I was very concerned and anxious about my missing memories. I remember always feeling anxious, and even in college I worried more than any of my friends. Although I was quiet and shy, I did have friends, dated, and even went to parties but didn't enjoy them much. Alcohol made me feel weird, and I really didn't like the effects of it, so I didn't drink any more than I had to in order to fit in. I dated some, but rarely anyone more than a few times—that is, until I met the woman who became my wife. She was calm, friendly, and accepted me for who I was—no pressure, no problems—which is why I am in love with her.

I researched the Internet for hints about the cause of my missing memories but quickly found that most websites only wanted to sell me something that would "fix my problems forever." Finally, I made an appointment with my family doctor and explained what was happening to me. She said it was a particular type of amnesia and wasn't necessarily a serious problem. After running several tests, she told me that there was nothing serious but that she was referring me to a neurologist for a second opinion.

At this point, I was becoming more anxious. Did I have a type of brain disease? Was I going to die? The neurologist quickly put me at ease, saying that it was unlikely anything serious would be found. He conducted several tests and reported to me that neurologically I was in great shape and that the problem must be psychological. He referred me to a psychologist who works with amnesia problems. Although I was embarrassed to tell my wife, she was so relieved that she began to cry. "I know this is something you can fix," she said. "I am so proud of you for trying to find some answers. You take care of yourself now, and let the kids and me take care of everything else."

Well, that did it; she had taken away all of my excuses. I made an appointment with the psychologist, and we started to work on my problem. I was quite comfortable with him asking me a few questions and then just letting me talk. I felt better after seeing him only one time because I felt that I was on the right track. I even looked forward to my next visit.

After a few visits, he discussed psychogenic amnesia with me and suggested that it was probably related to the abuse I had experienced as a child. He told me that this problem was typically responsive to psychotherapy but that progress would not be easy. He suggested that I also see a psychiatrist, a doctor he knew who could prescribe medication for my anxiety, which at this time was becoming worse; I was glad to take his advice. The psychiatrist was very businesslike and got right to the point but was also very helpful and reassuring. She prescribed medications to control the symptoms of anxiety but warned me that medicine wasn't a cure for my memory loss. She also stressed that I had to continue with psychotherapy even after I started to feel better.

At first it was exciting to discover answers to problems that had been plaguing me forever. The medication I was taking helped me get through each day and do what I needed to do. But it was very difficult to dredge up old, hurtful memories. They felt like weights that had been pushing down on me all my life and had to be removed one at a time. The more I remembered, the angrier I felt. The psychologist said this is normal and healthy and that we needed to work through it together. He also told me that I couldn't hide from the memories any longer because it would cause the amnesia and anxiety to flourish. I didn't like feeling angry but understood why I had to continue working through it. I seriously hated what my father did to me and supposed that someday I might find a way to either forgive him or at least accept that what he did was the result of his being seriously messed up. I was not even close to being able to do that. I was also angry with my mother, because I believed that she should have done something and didn't. However, now I realize that she, too, was a victim as much as I and that she will always live with the guilt of not protecting her children. I have yet to talk to her about it, but someday I will tell her that I understand and don't blame her for anything.

I am pleased to report that my life is moving in a good direction, and every day seems a little better. My psychiatrist says that I won't be taking medication forever but that I need to stay on it for now, and I continue to take her advice. My psychologist tells me that he expects me to make a full recovery, that the anxiety will not be the problem that it is today, and that I should recover some or even most of my lost memories. He stresses that I need to deal with anxiety-producing situations with new tools, such as stress management, being more assertive, and learning to recognize anger as it begins to appear. I didn't think I had a problem with anger, but he said that it is my primary issue. I have suppressed and repressed the anger for so long that I can no longer recognize it, which means that it never disappears, even when it isn't noticeable. It all sounds logical and I guess he's right, but I am not quite sure how it works.

Life at home is much better, and I am able to do more with my wife and children. They seem more relaxed and happier since I have been making progress. My wife's doctor told her that she should be working with someone on stress management, too, because it would be helpful for her fibromyalgia. She sees a different psychologist to work on her own issues. Although life isn't perfect, I feel like I now have a life. I didn't realize it, but for a long time I had been a spectator of my own life. Also, we have planned our first family vacation to visit my brother in Colorado, and the kids are ecstatic.

My advice to those who are struggling with life's challenges is to be open to seeing a professional to help you find answers. Life is too short to struggle on your own.

CASE 3: CHERI, 35-YEAR-OLD DIVORCED WOMAN WITH ONE DAUGHTER

Where to begin? Well, I am always a nervous wreck and am afraid of almost everything. I worry incessantly and have panic attacks that scare me to death. The only thing that is worse than a panic attack is the constant fear that I am going to have a panic attack. If that sounds crazy, believe me, it is.

My mother always said that I was high strung, even as a child. I remember being scared and worrying most of the time. I never stayed over at other people's homes and didn't like going to parties. I was nervous whenever we traveled, and if I was in the car more than 15 minutes, I would panic and often demand that my parents return home. Many times I made them take me home sooner than we had planned. I now know that I was probably having panic attacks, but I didn't know it then. Even if I did, it would not have changed anything. I didn't have the attacks often as a child, but it was terrifying when they occurred. No one understood what was happening, especially me. Since each attack eventually subsided, my folks seemed to think that I was making them up to get attention or to get my own way. When I was finally old enough to stay at home myself, they didn't bother to take me at all.

Maybe the fear of traveling goes back to a serious car accident that momma had when I was five years old and sitting in the back seat. Momma did not have her seat belt on and hit her head on the windshield and was knocked out cold. She had a serious concussion and a neck injury that required wearing a neck brace for several months. I had a broken leg and some bumps and bruises. I remember never wanting to ride in the car before the crash, but this incident made it worse. When my folks thought I was sleeping, I sometimes heard them arguing (usually after a few drinks, I suspect). Daddy would say to momma how stupid she was for causing the wreck and ask her how could she have done it.

I always seemed to need my parents' support and reassurance. Since they both drank in the evening, I could usually sit quietly with them and watch TV or listen to them talk. They seemed to like having me with them, so I would stay up as long possible. Of course, I was always tired the next morning, but even when I went to bed late, I was never able to fall asleep quickly. I just laid in bed thinking, worrying, and listening to the sounds in the house. I tried once to go into my parents' room when I was scared and couldn't sleep, but they got angry and sent me back to my room; I never did that again.

School was never easy for me because I was either in the nurse's office, home sick, or in class worrying and feeling scared. The school psychologist told my parents that he thought I had Attention Deficit Disorder (ADD) but not the hyperactive kind. Since I couldn't listen to and understand instructions being given, it seemed like I was unable to pay attention. Since I often didn't remember what I was told, they were convinced I had ADD. My parents and teachers now had an explanation for my behavior, and everyone seemed happy that the problem was solved. Since they no longer expected me to do well in school, much of the pressure was off of me, and I just floated along. My doctor prescribed ADD medication for me, but it only repressed my appetite to the point that I lost so much weight that I looked like a skinny little scarecrow. Taking me off the medication allowed me to gain the weight back. Next, I saw a counselor who was supposed to help me with the ADD, but all she did was let me color and draw pictures; she didn't really help me at all. As an adult I read about ADD and I don't think that I have ever had ADD at all. Personally, I believe anxiety has always been the main issue for me.

I struggled through school and barely completed high school. I almost didn't graduate due to so many absences. I had to submit a note from my doctor saying that my absences were due to a psychological problem, even though he didn't know what the problem was. I finally saw a psychiatrist, who put me on a tranquilizer. He said that I suffered from an Anxiety Disorder and needed to be on medication. Taking the drug did make me feel more re-laxed and stopped the anxiety attacks, which was a big plus, but nothing else changed. I was still plagued with a lot of fears and still worried all of the time and couldn't go anyplace or do the things that other people my age seemed to do easily. I think that I was the only one in my family who suffered from anxiety. If you ask my parents, they will say that everyone else is just fine. My sister Chrissy is a little high strung but is fine, too. They talk like we are just a normal, average family, just your basic *Leave It to Beaver*, middle-class, regular family—more like the *Addams Family* if you ask me. My parents drank too much and didn't seem to care about each other, except to have a drink-ing buddy, and they rarely talked, except about what was on TV. My brother (three years older) was always in trouble—nothing terrible but always into something. In high school, he was using drugs and alcohol, but my folks wrote it off to "boys will be boys." He tried to get me to smoke some weed by saying it would relax and loosen me up, but I was too scared to do it.

In terms of other family members, momma said that grandma had been troubled all of her life. It sounded to me like depression, but I am not sure since she died when I was fairly young. The only time we saw other family members in those days was during the holidays. Since everyone was drinking and laughing, I couldn't tell what they were truly like. My cousins were either older or younger than me and none of them liked to play with me, so I usually stayed in my room when they visited.

I find it interesting that I was able to be married, but it was sort of a fluke. A boy from high school who seemed to like me, although I can't imagine why, would come by my house and, occasionally, I would gather the courage to see a movie with him. He called me "interesting" and said that he would always be there to take care of me. Following high school, he went to work for his father in their car repair shop, while I worked fast food, retail, and volun-teered at the church. I couldn't do jobs that required me to think on my feet and serve people. It was too stressful and never lasted more than a few days. I liked helping at the church because no one rushed me and they were all nice to me. However, my parents made it very clear to me that I needed to find a job to support myself.

My daddy had worked for General Electric for many years and pulled some strings to get me a job there as a clerk-typist. Going to work daily was one of the toughest things I had ever done. But after a while I became used to the office environment, and it became another safe place for me. In fact, I eventually felt more comfortable at work than I did at home with my parents. They were arguing more often, my brother was in and out of trouble and jail, and I needed to move into my own apartment—which I did. A year later my boyfriend and I married, settled into our own place, and began what I had hoped would be a good life together.

A couple of years later we had a daughter, and I was absolutely thrilled. I felt as though my life was going to be normal. I still experienced anxiety, and when I went off of the medication while pregnant, the panic attacks returned. I began to isolate again, using the excuse that I was pregnant and couldn't do much. When the baby was tiny, I stayed at home for six weeks but soon had to return to work due to finances. My husband began going out often in the evenings and rarely spent time with me or our daughter. It became clear that he was cheating on me with more than one woman, and soon we were divorced, with me getting full custody of our daughter. He paid me child support and would take our daughter occasionally for a visit, but never for very long.

When my daughter entered school, new problems began; she wanted to have a normal life with friends and activities besides going with me to work, shopping, or staying home when that was all I could manage. I was back on medication again and began therapy with someone who was supportive and nice, but she didn't do much else for me. Other than the medication helping to reduce the anxiety, I still felt the same and wasn't getting any better.

I met a nice, understanding man at work who was about 15 years older than me and we were eventually married. My daughter didn't like him or the attention that I gave him and resented any time I spent with him. The marriage lasted 18 months before he finally had had enough of my daughter and me. Once again I was lonely, isolated, and anxious.

My daughter is now in high school, and I am happy to say that she is not at all like me. She is outgoing, fun, actively involved in school, a good student, and hopes to go to college. She brings friends over to the house and has a nice, polite boyfriend. They sometimes go to parties but usually just go to his house or ours to watch movies. My daughter has given up on me and never asks me to take her anywhere. I have never taken her on a vacation, although I did ask her father once if he would take her, but he said he was too busy. He rarely sees her anymore, and she doesn't seem to care one way or the other.

I wish that I could report that things are getting better, but they aren't. My daughter is going to be fine, and I am totally supportive of her going to college. Her father has stepped up to pay his share of her expenses, and I am so glad this won't be a problem—she deserves a better life than we have given to her up to this point.

I am still taking medication and found another therapist, although he isn't doing much for me either. He has some weird ideas about therapy and has me doing stuff that doesn't make much sense to me, but he assures me that if I get in touch with my inner energies and release them from my spiritual prison, I can shake the bonds of anxiety and fly free and happy into the future. Sounds good, but I have yet to see any flying or anything in the way of results. This probably explains why he has a degree in some alternative profession and does not have a state license. I will try this for a while and then maybe try to find someone a little more conventional. What I have read tells me that there are some good treatments for anxiety and panic attacks, but I have yet to find one. My daughter will be off to college in a couple of years, and then I am going to do whatever it takes to put this anxiety behind me. I may be miserable now, but I am not ready to give up. Please hope and pray for me—it is my turn to have a life, too.

SUMMARY

Each story represents a number of different but real people who have shared their pain and struggles while dealing with anxiety. No two stories are alike, and no two patients are the same. As you read more about anxiety and Anxiety Disorders, imagine waking up each morning knowing that another anxiety-filled day is ahead of you and hoping that it won't be too bad. The people who struggle with these disorders often have far more strength than is apparent, and living each day with the kinds of symptoms they must manage is quite impressive.

3

The Distribution and Effects of Anxiety Disorders: Costs, Gender, Age, and Specific Groups

> Neither comprehension nor learning can take place in an atmosphere of anxiety.
>
> —Rose F. Kennedy, mother of President John F. Kennedy

Each of us has experienced feelings of anxiety at some time, but, although it is possible for anyone to develop an Anxiety Disorder, most do not. Anxiety Disorders affect up to 26.9 million Americans at some point in their lives, and the costs of these disorders run about $46.6 billion per year, which accounts for 31.5 percent of total expenditures on mental illness in the United States. Of particular concern is that less than 25 percent of expenses associated with Anxiety Disorders have to do with medical or psychological treatments, while more than 75 percent reflect the patients' and families' lost income and reduced productivity.[1]

Anxiety Disorders significantly impact patients' daily lives as well patients' families, friends, and workplaces. The financial impact on the community is also quite significant. Costs for Anxiety Disorders in other industrialized Western countries are relatively the same, and it is likely that similar patterns and expenses exist throughout the world, although there is far less information available about the less developed areas. Within the United States, estimates of those who are diagnosed with and treated for Anxiety Disorders are quite low; for example, only 50 percent of patients will be accurately diagnosed with an Anxiety Disorder by their primary care physicians, and only 50 percent of those will actually receive appropriate treatment. If these estimates are even close to being accurate, then less than 25 percent of those suffering from Anxiety Disorders in the United States receive adequate treatment at the primary care level, and this number is most assuredly even lower in other areas of the world.[2]

Anxiety Disorders are the most commonly diagnosed psychiatric illnesses (25%), with Depression (17%) as the next most prevalent condition. Over the course of a lifetime, the occurrence rate for Anxiety Disorders in men is 19.2 percent and in women 30.5 percent.[2] Approximately 2 of every 10 men and 3 of every 10 women will develop an Anxiety Disorder during their life; in 1990 dollars that projects to about $1,542 annually per patient, with 88 percent of that cost due to lost productivity. Two specific Anxiety Disorders, Posttraumatic Stress Disorder (PTSD) and Panic Disorder, have the highest rate of mental health and medical service use of any psychiatric illnesses.[3] The majority of calculated expenses associated with Anxiety Disorders could be dramatically reduced if more time and resources were focused on accurately diagnosing and treating patients sooner. Although increased finances would need to be directed into treatment delivery, in the long run the non-treatment losses (e.g., family, friends, jobs) and the length of a course of treatment would significantly decrease.

GENDER AND ANXIETY DISORDERS

Women and Anxiety

Women of all ages suffer from Anxiety Disorders and Depression more frequently than do men. Symptoms in women do not always manifest the same in women as they do in men, and symptoms can also vary as a function of age. Many believe, although erroneously, that gender is a significant risk factor for developing an Anxiety Disorder and must be carefully considered in prevention and intervention programs.[4] In one study, 19 percent of women reported significant symptoms of anxiety that were intrusive to activities of daily living, such as bathing, dressing, walking, lifting, and doing light housework.[5] Women with Anxiety Disorders may decide to curtail their activities due to a feeling of being at risk or due to physical symptoms, such as feeling shaky; they feel as though they may be unable to function normally.[5] Research indicates that Anxiety Disorders are frequently a component of the diagnoses for those who qualify for disability benefits due to their inability to work regularly to support themselves.

The reasons for women being diagnosed and treated more frequently for Anxiety Disorders are numerous and not simple. Some research suggests that fluctuations in the levels of female reproductive hormones and cycles may have an effect on anxiety. While it is true that during Pre-Menstrual Syndrome, Pre-Menstrual Dysphoric Disorder, and menopause, women are more likely to experience anxiety and to develop a diagnosable Anxiety Disorder, varying hormone levels are not the only reasons. Women tend also to be more prone to anxiety for a variety of biological, psychological, and cultural factors, as will be discussed further in chapter 4. For example, research suggests that psychological factors, such as women being less assertive or society being more accepting of women expressing their fears, can increase the likelihood of women developing anxiety (or acknowledging it) more often than men. Also, there seems to be a genetic role that affects the probability of an Anxiety Disorder developing, although this is not yet fully understood.[6] While most research has been conducted in the United States and Western Europe, one's gender is a significant element noted while studying health inequities across all developing countries and has a strong influence over the amount of control that men and women can exercise over the determinants of their own health, including the economic resources and social status, which provide differential access to care and treatment.[7]

Men and Anxiety

Although there is no single or simple explanation for it, men are less likely to be diagnosed with an Anxiety Disorder than are women. Significant numbers of men do experience problems with anxiety, but they often choose not to seek help due to the stigma of having a condition that implies weakness or frailty. Frequently, professionals do not recognize symptoms of anxiety in men patients because the complaints reported are more often physical and not feelings of anxiety or fear. Typically, men who are brought to an emergency room with symptoms of a panic attack are more likely to be suspected of having a heart attack than being acutely anxious, although the opposite is true for women.[6] Men are more likely to self medicate with alcohol and/or drugs, which can mask or distort symptoms of anxiety and lead to misdiagnoses.[8] Men also display different symptom patterns from women when experiencing anxiety; for example, it is far more likely that women who suffer from Anxiety or Panic Disorder will develop Agoraphobia (the fear of going out to places among strangers), while men are not as likely to experience agoraphobia.[9] It is difficult to determine the specific differences between men and women who suffer from Anxiety Disorders, because women seek treatment for these conditions more often than men,[6] which means there are fewer untreated women with Anxiety Disorders and less data collected on men.

One interesting study shows noticeable gender differences in Anxiety Disorder patients among urban and metropolitan people but not among those in rural areas. In fact, rural men more often report Mood and Anxiety Disorders than urban men. In trying to understand this phenomenon, it is believed that rural men may be more prone to Anxiety and Depressive Disorders because they lack opportunities for important resources such as steady, high-paying jobs and often live under a constant financial strain. This finding is most noticeable among white men, who comprise the majority of rural residents.[10] It is also true that men in rural areas often do not have appropriate mental health services available, and this, of course, is also true of women in rural regions.

Gender differences among other types of Anxiety Disorder patients produce interesting patterns as well. For example, women with PTSD show a curvilinear pattern of lifetime exposure to trauma, while men show a linear increase. This means that women experience various rates of exposure to trauma at differing ages, while men tend to show an increase in exposure to traumatic events over time.[11] The most common explanation for this is exposure to combat trauma. However, one recent study found that PTSD symptoms in professional career firefighters was positively correlated with their age.[12] As people get older (in this case, firefighters), they tend to report more PTSD symptoms. This implies that the experience of professional firefighters over time produces a cumulative psychological impact, and this probably applies to police and military personnel as well—all jobs traditionally held by men. Therefore, one reason why men tend to show a linear increase in exposure to trauma is that they more often work in areas and professions where continuing and cumulative exposure to traumatic events occurs.

No clear-cut explanations account for the variety of experiences and symptoms found between men and women. Some biological differences may predispose women to having anxiety-related problems, but this alone is not an adequate explanation. Socialization and related psychological issues also affect a woman's chances of developing an Anxiety Disorder in most cultures. If we consider all of the risk factors for developing Anxiety Disorders—biological, psychological, social, cultural, and others—we can conclude that, the *more* and/or *more severe* risk factors to which a person is exposed, the greater the chance that a person will develop a disorder. Women, in general, tend to have more risk factors and are, therefore, more likely to develop Anxiety Disorders, even when we control for the frequency of reporting differences between the sexes. One encouraging study reports that men and women patients with anxiety, who were followed over a five-year period, both showed 39 percent remission rates (reporting no symptoms of the disorder) following treatment.[9] This statistic demonstrates that men are just as likely as women to improve following treatment and, therefore, should seek help when needed.

AGE AND ANXIETY

Children and Teens and Anxiety

Specific fears and social fears are common among children when they are young, and most will outgrow them as they mature. Specific and social phobias are diagnosed in children only when symptoms have been present for at least six months.[13] while the transient fears, common to many children, would not be diagnosed as a disorder unless they did not diminish within six months. Diagnostically, it is more common for children to be diagnosed with Oppositional Defiant Disorder and Attention Deficit Hyperactivity Disorder than Anxiety Disorder, but many children studied in a community sample of four-year-olds were found to have problems with anxiety, although it was usually not the most pressing problem they were experiencing.[14] Other than Separation Anxiety Disorder, which is specific to children, youngsters experience the same types of Anxiety Disorders as do adults, such as Generalized Anxiety Disorder, Panic Disorder, Specific and Social Phobias, Obsessive-Compulsive Disorder, Posttraumatic and Acute Stress Disorders, and Agoraphobia. These disorders are discussed more fully in chapters 5 and 6.

One of the differences between children and adults, when it comes to fears and phobias, is that children are less likely to recognize that their fears are excessive or unrealistic.[15] For many children, their fears are associated with school and school-related activities, and it is not uncommon for children to report being fearful of changing clothes in gym class, eating in the cafeteria, speaking in front of the class, and other typical school activities. It is also not unusual for children to feign illness in order to stay at home and avoid the situations that frighten them.

The reported differences between boys and girls with respect to phobias and fears are mixed, but most children will significantly improve with treatment. Some researchers have found no sex differences in phobias at all,[16] but others have found that girls experience more phobias than boys.[17] One study that followed a group of children over a three- to four-year period found that 70 percent of those with Specific Phobia recovered, and 86 percent with Social Phobia recovered; this appears to be true for both boys and girls.[18]

Diagnosing Anxiety Disorders in children is challenging because many of their symptoms are somatic (physical) in nature. One study found that 96 percent of children with Anxiety Disorders presented with physical symptoms, each having an average of six different physical symptoms. The most common were restlessness (74%), stomachaches (70%), blushing (50%), palpitations, (48%), muscle tension (45%), sweating (45%), and trembling/shaking (43%). Boys and girls presented approximately the same number of symptoms, although boys tended to report stomachaches and chest pains more frequently than girls, and older children typically reported more symptoms than younger ones. Symptom patterns varied slightly between types of Anxiety Disorders, but treatment effectively reduced symptoms in all of the different conditions.[19]

When comparing children who suffer from the same disorders, other than Anxiety Disorder, it appears that those who also experience anxiety in addition to their other problems have more frequently experienced negative life events.[20] Thus, it is likely that these children develop Anxiety Disorders at a higher rate due to actually living in a stressful environment fraught with numerous, negative events and not simply that negative interpretations of these events have resulted from filtering them through a child's haze of anxiety. Children with a condition called Generalized Anxiety Disorder (GAD), which is characterized by general and free-floating anxiety, worry more than other children about negative circumstances in their lives, and they appear to experience more negative events during their short lives than others of the same age. Thus, not only do they worry more, but they actually seem to have more negative things to worry about as well.

In teens the rate of Anxiety Disorders is relatively high, with 2.8 percent presenting significant symptoms of anxiety. It is difficult to determine specific causal factors for anxiety in teens, but, as with younger children, teens with anxiety symptoms showed higher rates of stress, particularly when there was an adverse family context.[21] Interestingly, teens with Anxiety Disorders report less peer contact than other teens, which may be due to anxiety causing them to avoid contact with others, especially when in larger groups.[22] Although anxious teens may intentionally avoid peer contact and conflict, peer conflict probably is not the major source of the anxiety that they are experiencing. This does not mean that youngsters do not experience anxiety due to fears or concerns about peers, but rather that Anxiety Disorders are not simply caused by peer contact or conflict. The avoidance of peers is probably more a symptom of anxiety than the cause of the Anxiety Disorder.

Another study examined anxiety sensitivity in adolescents, which refers to the tendency to experience anxiety more frequently and intensely. In both African American and white youths, anxiety sensitivity is more likely to be associated with the subsequent development of Panic Disorder.[23] In fact, teens who are very sensitive to anxiety are more likely to experience panic symptoms later—even if they do not have them when first evaluated. If early-onset panic symptoms are detected and controlled through treatment, anxiety sensitivity does not predict an increase in panic symptoms later and is less likely to cause problems in the future.[23] Therefore, using anxiety sensitivity as a risk factor can help professionals identify youths who are at risk for developing Anxiety Disorders and then treating them early enough to reduce the need for treatment later.

In college students, the patterns in Anxiety Disorders are similar to those in older teens and younger adults. As might be anticipated, anxiety problems will negatively affect interpersonal relations, emotional regulation, and personal adult attachment. The more anxiety problems that college students experience, the more difficulties they will have in school and with social activities.[24] One advantage for college students is the availability of an on-campus student health center or a university (college) counseling center. Students, who are reluctant to tell their parents about a problem or to seek advice privately, can go to a campus counseling or health center for help dealing with anxiety. One additional risk for college students is the easy access to alcohol and drugs as a way of coping with their anxiety instead of, or in addition to, seeking treatment.

As mentioned earlier, one of the difficult realities of diagnosing and treating Anxiety Disorders is the frequency of patients having comorbidities (other conditions), and in youths with Anxiety Disorders, comorbidities are the rule, not the exception. In one encouraging study, the presence of comorbidities did not negatively affect treatment outcomes for anxiety.[25] A common symptom of Anxiety Disorder in children and youths is the presence of Sleep-Related Problems (SRPs). Although sometimes considered a comorbid condition, SRPs are more often a direct result of the Anxiety Disorder and are almost always present. For example, 98 percent of youth with Generalized Anxiety Disorder, 97 percent with Separation Anxiety, and 90 percent with Social Anxiety had at least one SRP, and 55 percent had three or more. SRPs were also significant predictors of anxiety severity and of family functioning in the home. The good news was that following eight weeks of treatment with fluvoxamine (a selective serotonin reuptake inhibitor antidepressant) teen patients significantly improved and reported fewer SRPs.[26] It is clear that SRPs are not a cause of Anxiety Disorders, nor are they typically a comorbid condition, but rather they are symptoms of the Anxiety Disorder and will decrease or disappear when the Anxiety Disorder is treated. That does not mean that a teen who has an Anxiety Disorder *cannot* have a primary SRP, but most frequently sleep problems are secondary to the anxiety in youngsters with Anxiety Disorders.

Another significant comorbid condition for children and teens with Anxiety Disorder is an Autistic Spectrum Disorder (ASD)—a serious type of Developmental Disorder that includes Autism, Asperger's Syndrome, and Pervasive Developmental Disorder—and children with an ASD have a higher risk of developing an Anxiety Disorder. The symptoms of anxiety in children with ASD are similar to those who do not have ASD, impacting their lives in similar ways, but ASDs tend to create more challenges in dealing with difficult developmental issues. We treat Anxiety Disorder in children with an ASD in a similar manner as children without ASD, since ASD children do not seem to experience serious fears more frequently than do other children, nor does having an ASD cause the Anxiety Disorder itself to worsen.[27]

Diagnosing and Treating Children and Teens

It is not uncommon for Anxiety Disorders in children to go unrecognized or be written off as some other problem. For example, parents will often hear advice such as, "Ignore it; don't worry—they will grow out of it," and this is often the case. Sometimes clinicians do not recognize that Anxiety Disorders among children can be related to adult Anxiety Disorders. Also, children with Anxiety Disorders can self-limit their own exposures to age-appropriate situations, which could negatively affect their development if the Anxiety Disorders are not treated.[28] Therefore, it is important that childhood Anxiety Disorders be treated early and effectively. Recent studies indicate that most children with Anxiety Disorders are not receiving appropriate treatment, and lack of care will affect the child's development, happiness, and future health.[28]

Treatments that are endorsed by mental health professionals and that are available to children and teens with Anxiety Disorders include medications combined with Cognitive-behavioral therapy (CBT). However, youths and their parents are often initially less accepting of these types of treatments and are more likely to embrace informal supportive gestures such as family, friends, and support groups as treatment alternatives for Anxiety Disorders.[29] Parents are frequently reluctant to approve medication and CBT, because their acceptance of such treatments is a formal admission that their child does not simply have a minor problem that they will eventually outgrow, and they often harbor concerns about the risks of taking medications. Professionals must educate patients, friends, and families about the benefits of early recognition and treatment and encourage questions and discussions regarding medication risks and myths *in the presence of the young patient.*

Support and interventions offered by family and friends to patients dealing with anxiety problems can be helpful, but these are not a substitute for professional treatment. However, family involvement can be integrated into a treatment or prevention program in ways that can be very beneficial. One imaginative program involved children and families in a Coping and Promoting Strength Program (CPSP), while others were placed in a waitlist control group and were offered the option to enter the program one year later. The children chosen for the program were deemed high risk for Anxiety Disorders because their parents had met a wide range of criteria for a variety of Anxiety Disorders. After one year, 30 percent of the waitlist group developed an Anxiety Disorder, while no one in the CPSP group developed one, which highlights the importance of early detection and treatment of children with anxiety problems. Clearly, early anxiety symptoms in children and teens are key risk factors for developing Anxiety Disorders as adults, and family-based prevention programs can be an effective way to reduce the incidence of adult anxiety problems.[30]

Anxiety Disorders in the Elderly

Although depression is considered a common problem among the elderly, anxiety is more frequently challenging and affects between 10 percent and

24 percent of older individuals, depending on the study. One difficulty in detecting and diagnosing anxiety problems in the elderly is that they often report physical rather than cognitive symptoms of anxiety. Clinicians who are screening for anxiety problems in the elderly need to focus more on the physical symptoms when considering a diagnosis.[31]

Although Generalized Anxiety Disorder, one of the most common Anxiety Disorders, is less prevalent in older adults than in other age groups, it is still a significant and regular problem among the elderly.[32] In older patients, anxiety is associated with diminished well-being and increased disability, and while the use of general health services is increased among elderly anxiety sufferers, the commitment to appropriate care is typically low. This could be the result of a lack of understanding about Anxiety Disorder but is more likely due to a minimal number of valid diagnoses and treatment referrals. Providers sometimes consider symptoms of anxiety in the elderly an understandable reaction to life's frequent negative events in this age group, but the symptoms experienced are virtually the same as others who suffer from Anxiety Disorders and who have experienced few negative life events.[33] Regardless of the source of the anxiety, the elderly are deserving of and can benefit from effective treatment.

The Longitudinal Aging Study Amsterdam (LASA) examined a community sample of more than three thousand older adults and found that anxiety is relatively common in later life. These people, who were not identified as patients, had an overall prevalence rate for Anxiety Disorders of 10.2 percent. The most common disorder was GAD (7.3%), followed by Phobic Disorder (3.1%), and Panic Disorder (1.0%). The researchers also found that the aging process itself did not impact the frequency of Anxiety Disorders but that many of life's events did make the elderly more vulnerable. For example, being a woman, having lower education levels, experiencing negative events during World War II, and having an external locus of control were all factors that predisposed people to develop an Anxiety Disorder.[34] Having an external locus of control means that people with this trait feel that the control of events that are important to them come from outside of themselves (e.g., fate, luck, other people). A study by DeBeurs et al. found that the most stressful life event that may lead to anxiety problems is the death of a spouse.[35] The LASA study also found that stress factors such as a recent family loss or chronic physical illness or pain play a role in the development of Anxiety Disorders in older adults.[34]

Although anxiety is a common and debilitating problem in the elderly, it is frequently overlooked or dismissed by providers, family, and friends. In addition, 90 percent of the elderly with Anxiety Disorders suffer from at least one comorbid psychological problem, which increases their risk of physical disability, memory problems, a reduced quality of life, and even death.[36] Diagnosing Anxiety Disorders in the elderly is more challenging, because the symptoms are usually physical and are often vague and difficult to differentiate from other physical or psychological problems. Further, anxiety can exacerbate the symptoms of other medical disorders, making them more difficult to treat. Further complicating treatment, an older person with Anxiety Disorder who develops a new medical problem faces the additional challenge of feeling increased anxiety about the new medical diagnosis and its treatment.[36]

Anxiety Disorders in older people can and should be treated, although treatment response and follow-through is lower than in other age groups due to several factors.[36] First, people from older generations are generally less aware of psychological issues and are more likely to blame their anxiety symptoms on an illness or physical condition. Second, transportation issues and financial concerns may present problems in seeking a location for treatment. Third, taking medication for an Anxiety Disorder, which is often used as the first line of treatment, presents several possible problems for the elderly. Medications are often not as effective in older people, and, because they have lower metabolic rates, the elderly are more likely to experience negative side effects and are less likely to tolerate a therapeutic dosage level. Some of the side effects, such as drowsiness and impaired balance and cognitive function, can be dangerous. In general, older people are taking more and different types of medications, and these may interact with the psychotropic (psychiatric) drugs, producing unwanted side effects. However, the elderly tend to respond well to psychotherapy, and some professionals feel that a low-dose medication coupled with psychotherapy is the best treatment for the elderly with anxiety problems. Cognitive-behavioral therapy is considered by most practitioners as the first line of treatment for Anxiety Disorders in the elderly.[36] While the combination of CBT and medication works well for both the general population and for elderly patients with Anxiety and Panic Disorders, further analysis revealed that the improvement was largely due to the CBT rather than medications.[37]

Clearly, Anxiety Disorders are common and problematic among the elderly, but research on the course and treatment lags well behind research on Depression and Dementia. We used to think that anxiety problems decreased with age, but obviously this is not true. Anxiety Disorders are as common in older adults as they are in other age groups, although the symptoms present somewhat differently. Typically, the elderly suffer from both Anxiety and Depression, and women with less education are at increased risk for developing both problems. Older persons with Anxiety Disorder probably suffered from anxiety when they were younger, but often the complexities of aging elicit an Anxiety Disorder and establish more obvious symptoms.

Treatment of Anxiety in the Elderly

Treatment of Anxiety Disorders in the elderly usually begins with the primary care physician and involves the prescribing of antidepressant medications (usually the selective serotonin reuptake inhibitors and serotonin-norepinephrine reuptake inhibitors) as the first line of medication treatment; however, as mentioned above, CBT is also very effective with the elderly. A good therapeutic alliance between the primary care physician, mental health and medical specialists, the patient, and the family is the key to effective treatment.[6]

Anxiety Disorder is considered to be a Diathesis-Stress Disorder; a *diathesis* is a predisposition to developing a particular condition due to genetics, one's constitution, early learning or experiences, or other factors. The stress portion of the equation can be experiences of certain factors within the environment and/or experiences from a person's past. The logic of the diathesis-stress model is that someone who possesses certain risk factors and who reports critical/serious life experiences is more likely to develop the disorder in question. The presence of these risk factors should alert treating professionals to screen for Anxiety Disorders on a regular basis and to begin treatment early, thus improving the likelihood for success.

Research worldwide on Depression in the elderly is consistent with studies done in the United States, and we expect similar results for Anxiety Disorders. One study looked at mental health problems in the elderly in a primary care setting in the province of Huesca, Spain.[38] At the time of assessment, about 46.1 percent of the patients presented with psychiatric symptoms, and anxiety was the second most frequently reported condition (15.7%) behind cognitive impairment (16.4%); women were almost twice as likely as men to have psychiatric symptoms. The factors related to psychiatric symptoms were age, severity of physical illness, poor social support, and previous psychiatric comorbidity. Since only 29 percent of patients in this sample had a previous diagnosis of a psychiatric illness, it is clear that many of these patients had not been appropriately diagnosed at the primary care level. This demonstrates the need for the improved training of professionals to recognize and diagnose mental illness at the primary care level; this is consistent with findings in the United States, particularly for patients who fall outside the typical majority, including older adults.

RACE, ETHNICITY, AND ANXIETY DISORDERS

There is evidence of anxiety and fear-based psychological problems within all cultures. They may be identified by different names or be perceived differently, and the availability of care may be quite different, but no culture is immune. This makes understanding and comparing anxiety among cultures both challenging and complex, since behavior in one culture might be indicative of anxiety, but in another it may mean something quite different.

In the United States, the lack of eye contact while speaking may be interpreted as a lack of assertiveness or indicative of anxiety or dishonesty. However, among Mexican Americans and among the Japanese, the lack of eye contact is considered a sign of respect. Smiling at someone in the United States might convey acceptance or comfort, but in Japan a smile is a sign of embarrassment or discomfort.[39] Even the manner of speech or the number of words used, as well as the tonal and volume aspects of speech, can imply different meanings to peoples from other cultures. White Americans are typically uncomfortable with silence, but the British and Arabs use silence for privacy, and other cultural groups employ silence as a sign of respect or an indication of agreement. Asians typically speak more quietly than Americans, who speak more softly than many from Arab countries.[15] Clearly, when trying to understand a person's behavior, it is important to be knowledgeable of cultural differences so an accurate assessment is achieved.

African Americans and Anxiety

African Americans experience Anxiety Disorders in different patterns, and their access to treatment is not generally equal to that of the white population. As with other groups, the stigma of mental illness prevents some African Americans from seeking care, even those who have adequate health insurance. But the disturbing fact that over 25 percent of African Americans do not have health insurance is significant as well. Only one-third of African Americans who need care for Anxiety Disorders receive it, and they are more likely to terminate treatment prematurely. Further, African Americans are more likely to receive temporary or inadequate mental health treatment at the primary care level, which is one reason why they are overrepresented in emergency room visits and inpatient mental health hospitalizations. Psychological treatments are as effective and successful as with white patients, but African Americans rarely seek out a mental health professional and thus typically do not receive needed treatment.[40]

The types of Anxiety Disorders for which African American patients do receive treatment tend to be different from the disorders reported by white patients. The Epidemiologic Catchment Area study of the National Institute of Mental Health found that the lifetime prevalence rates of Simple Phobia and Agoraphobia were significantly higher among African Americans than other groups and that racial differences in frequency rates did not exist with Panic Disorder or Anxiety Disorders in general.[41]

Some professionals believe that significant racial differences in help-seeking behaviors and symptom presentation may be responsible for underrecognition and misdiagnosis of Anxiety Disorders among African American patients in outpatient mental health settings. In the primary care setting, African Americans more often report physical symptoms of Anxiety Disorders and also present different patterns of comorbidity. Even when demographic and socioeconomic status (SES) are held constant, the racial differences for problems such as Phobias still remain, strongly indicating that being an African American is one of the risk factors for Phobias in addition to being female, young, and having lower educational attainment.[42]

Although the rate of Panic Disorder among African Americans and whites is similar, African Americans with Panic Disorder report more intense fears of dying or feelings of "going crazy," higher levels of numbing and tingling in their extremities, and higher rates of comorbid PTSD and Depression than white patients. They also tend to use different coping strategies (e.g., counting one's blessings), show less self-blame, and are more dissatisfied with the availability of social supports than whites.[43]

When examining the rates of Anxiety Disorders within different racial groups, it is important to recognize that patients exhibit multiple risk factors as well as differing patterns of comorbidities and to consider the whole picture. Many people over the age of 65 who are evaluated for Anxiety or Depression are likely to show patterns of alcohol misuse, and about 59 percent are minorities. In contrast to minimal treatment available at the primary care level, an integrated care setting that offers professional services in different specialties, such as alcohol and drug abuse counseling, typically provides much more responsive and coordinated care.[44] This is particularly important for minorities, such as African Americans, who are less frequently referred to specialists for mental health care.

Adequately diagnosing and treating Anxiety Disorders in all minority groups must be a priority and certainly among African Americans, for whom treatment rarely reaches threshold for attaining good clinical outcomes.[44] A better understanding of the differences in symptom presentation and treatment options is critical in order to deal more effectively with these highly treatable conditions. In contract, one study concluded that there are no real differences between white and African American patients with respect to Anxiety Disorders in general and no differences in the functional disability associated with them.[41] Still, there are many variations in the diagnosis and treatment of these conditions between the two groups, and it is obvious that with appropriate and adequate care, African Americans demonstrate the same rates of improvement and cures as do white people suffering from similar disorders.

Asian Americans and Anxiety

The literature on anxiety has not focused on Asian Americans, but, as a rapidly increasing cultural group that is presently underserved, we need to learn more about their mental health needs, particularly of older Asian Americans.[45] Asian Americans scored higher on measures of Depression and Social Anxiety and reported higher levels of distress than white Americans, with recent immigrants showing the highest levels of distress and demonstrating that ethnicity is related to Social Anxiety.[46] It is also true that Asian Americans are under represented among mental health professionals.

Growing literature supports the theory that ethnic differences affect rates of Social Anxiety, and studies of college students consistently have reported that Asian American students show higher levels of Social Anxiety than do European American students. Interestingly, some cross-cultural data suggest that shyness and Social Anxiety can be consistent with a culture's socialization patterns and is considered normal within some Asian groups. However, other research suggests that the experience of Social Anxiety is associated with subjective distress and functional impairment in Asian Americans. These subjects are rarely discussed with friends, however, because Asian students are more concerned than their white colleagues with "losing face" and with trying to avoid negative evaluations by others.[47]

It appears that Asian American students are at significant risk for Anxiety Disorders and Depression due to immigrant/minority status, cultural stressors, and developmental factors. Other stressors such as academic problems, family pressure, and acculturation complicate the college experience for Asian Americans and can lead to increased difficulties. To fully appreciate the challenges Asian students face, unique cultural issues, including a high emphasis on family loyalty and the adherence to collectivist values, must be considered. Research has consistently found that Asian American college students report higher levels of Anxiety and Depression than do other students and are more frequently at risk for negative mental health outcomes, and this is compounded by parental pressure, academic pressure, and acculturation issues.[48]

Attention has recently focused upon Japanese Americans, with some interesting findings. Japanese Americans conceptualize anxiety by describing more depressive symptoms than anxiety symptoms, especially among older Japanese American patients, making it difficult to accurately diagnose Anxiety Disorders. Also, Japanese Americans tend to report more cognitive symptoms than the somatic symptoms we find with other minority groups and with Americans in general.[49] Specific Phobias and related conditions exist within each culture, including Japan, but sometimes these conditions appear differently or have a different name. For example, in Japan there is a condition known as *taijin kyôfu*, when people are obsessed with shame. The symptoms are similar to Social Phobia, including the fears of blushing, exhibiting improper facial expressions in front of others, shaking, and perspiring,[50] but is it really Social Phobia? Diagnostically, the answer is irrelevant since the symptoms would be treated similarly. But symptoms that are primarily shame-based would indicate the need for the treating professional to use a different treatment approach than with other patients.

Research in mental health regarding Asians rarely focuses on one specific Asian group, such as the Japanese or Koreans; instead, more than 40 distinctly different Asian ethnic groups are viewed, unfortunately, in most of the literature as one homogeneous group. Most studies have focused on East Asians, including the Japanese, Chinese, and Koreans, and have neglected Southeast Asians such as Indians, Pakistanis, Bangladeshis, Nepalese, and Sri Lankans. Asian American women are particularly underrepresented in the literature, even though the research consistently demonstrates that women worldwide are more at risk for anxiety and depression. Some studies have also found that coping styles and stress factors related to immigration and acculturation have been linked to Depression and Anxiety Disorders among East Asian American women and South Asian American women.[50]

Asian Americans combined with American Pacific Islanders comprise a group with the lowest level of utilization of mental health services for any ethnic population, most likely due to cultural stigma and family influence. It is also true that the poverty rates for this group are lower than the national poverty average.[40] Asian American students experience discrimination like many ethnic minorities and are at higher risk for state and trait anxiety as well as depression, suicidal ideation, and psychological distress. State anxiety is where a person is anxious because of a specific situation or state, whereas trait anxiety refers to anxiety that is generally prevalent in a person and carries across situations or conditions. As might be expected, the perception of discrimination by a person of an ethnic minority is the basis of his or her experienced stress and anxiety, and for Asian Americans and Pacific Islanders, these perceptions are directly related to frequent negative mental health outcomes.[51]

In summary, Anxiety Disorders, including Phobias, exist within all cultural groups, including Asians. Available research suggests that women suffer more frequently from Anxiety Disorders, but in many Asian and Middle Eastern countries, men are more likely to seek and receive treatment. For example, in Saudi Arabia and India, 80 percent of the patients seeking mental health treatment were men. Even in Japan, where women might be expected to have better access to mental health care, 60 percent of people diagnosed with *taijin kyôfu* were men.[15]

The Asian and foreign-born populations in the United States are growing, and these populations are garnering more notice in the research literature and in clinical settings. Because people from all cultures suffer from Anxiety Disorders, it is important to appreciate the ethnicity and cultural background of each patient prior to diagnosing and prescribing treatment. Cultural awareness and sensitivity are critical factors to providing reasonable, responsible, and appropriate mental health services.

Hispanic Americans and Anxiety

Like other minorities in the United States, Hispanics deal with ethnic-specific challenges with regard to social, medical, and mental health issues, including anxiety. Hispanics, like Asians, are not a homogeneous group and include people from many different countries and cultures. However, they tend to be grouped together statistically in most research and demographic analyses. Hispanic Americans have the lowest per capita income of any ethnic group and are less likely to have health insurance—in fact, they are twice as likely to be uninsured than whites. Although the 1990 census reported that 40 percent of Hispanics could not speak English, only a few mental health providers can speak Spanish. In general, Hispanic immigrants have a lower rate of mental illness than Hispanics born in the United States,[40] and this finding suggests that difficulties with acculturation, discrimination, and immigrant status are related to their mental health difficulties. One study found that, when Asian American and Hispanic students are brought to the attention of school authorities, the Hispanic students are far more likely to be accused of wrongdoing such as cheating or breaking the law than the Asian students, and they are more likely to experience these events as stressful—especially when suspicions are cast upon them more frequently and independently of any actual wrongdoing.[52]

An interesting phenomenon called the Latino Paradox refers to the consistent finding that the mental health status of lower-SES–Latino/as tends to be better than that of low-SES whites or low-SES African Americans and that the risk for mental health problems within minority groups increases with the years lived in the United States. But, as mentioned above, treating Hispanics as a homogeneous group is misleading since significant differences exist by area of origin and degree of acculturation. For example, Puerto Rican mothers and fathers are more likely to meet the criteria for Major Depression and Generalized Anxiety Disorder than Hispanics from any other area. In fact, Puerto Rican Americans are at greatest risk for Depression and Anxiety Disorders one year after the birth of a child, while Mexican Americans are at the lowest risk. The average risk of the two Hispanic groups taken together appears to be normal, but the differences between the cultural groups suggest that professionals could overlook a diagnosis of Anxiety Disorder or Depression due to being unfamiliar with each group's risk factors and symptoms.[52]

Native Americans and Alaskan Natives and Anxiety

As with other minority groups, there is minimal comprehensive and appropriate research on the mental health needs and issues for Native Americans and Alaskan Natives, and numerous challenges are not being adequately addressed. Past attempts to eradicate the culture of Native Americans have been associated with negative mental health consequences,[40] and even when intentions were good, the results were quite harmful. During the late 19th and early to mid-20th centuries in many Midwestern and Southwestern states, "Indian Schools" were created and intended to bring education, literacy, and economic self-reliance to the Native people. However, the education element also included the conversion to Christianity and an effort to stamp out Native religious beliefs. State governments also tried to get the Native American children to become like the white majority population, an effort believed by most whites to be positive. Largely, they succeeded in stripping the Natives of their spiritual beliefs, culture, sense of heritage, and the support they should have received from their tribal groups.

Native Americans and Alaskan Natives are significantly impoverished, with more than 25 percent living below the poverty level, and some studies found that negative mental health outcomes are related to their minority status and their financial and social hardships. Native American veterans of the Vietnam War suffered more PTSD and long-term alcohol abuse than did African Americans or Japanese Americans, and had few opportunities for the treatment they needed. While many people would prefer to see a professional from their own cultural background, there are only 101 Native American or Alaskan Native mental health professionals per 100,000 people, compared to 173 white mental health professionals per 100,000 whites. In 1996 there were only 20 psychiatrists of Native American or Alaskan Native heritage practicing in the United States. It is not surprising that many people in these groups seek advice from traditional healers within their own culture and, when available, combine it with conventional care.[40]

Summary

In some Native American languages, words for depression and anxiety do not even exist, but the suicide rate for Native American and Alaskan Native young men between the ages of 15 and 24 is two to three times higher than the national rate. Mental health needs are not being recognized or addressed, and adequate treatment is not being provided. Among Asian Americans and Pacific Islanders, the rate of mental illness is not that different from other Americans, but they have the lowest utilization rates of mental health services of any minority. Mexican-born Americans have a 25 percent rate of mental illness, while Mexicans born in the United States have a 48 percent rate—clearly a growing and serious problem.[40]

Culture affects the way people communicate and manifest their symptoms of mental illness, including Anxiety Disorders, as well as their choice of coping styles, family and community supports, and a willingness to seek treatment. Minorities are also overrepresented among the most vulnerable, high-need groups—such as the homeless and incarcerated persons—and these populations have a much higher rate of mental illness than people living "normally" in the community. Ample evidence demonstrates that the disability burden as a result of unmet or inadequately met mental health needs is disproportionately high for racial and ethnic minorities relative to whites[40]—this needs to be addressed in a serious and programmatic way.

HOMOSEXUAL GROUPS AND ANXIETY

Gay men and lesbian women are specific subgroups who have largely been ignored in the research, partially because they are not easy to recognize unless they identify themselves to treatment professionals. Data suggest, however, that levels of depression and anxiety in homosexual persons are substantially higher than in the heterosexual population.[53] Mood and Anxiety Disorders are more prevalent among those who have had one or more same-sex partners, including gay, lesbian, and bisexual individuals. Gay and bisexual men are 4.7 times more likely to be diagnosed with Panic Disorder than other men, and lesbian and bisexual women were more likely to be diagnosed with Generalized Anxiety Disorder than heterosexual women.[54]

One encouraging study found that those in the lesbian/gay/bisexual (LGB) community are more likely to access mental health services than the heterosexual population. Among gay and bisexual men, 85.3 percent received some type of mental health services compared with 45.2 percent of heterosexual men, and about 94 percent of lesbian and bisexual women accessed mental health services compared to 54 percent of heterosexual women.[54]

As might be expected, many feel their homosexual status is a significant issue when dealing with other people, and gay men report a greater fear of negative evaluation and social interaction anxiety as well as lower self-esteem than heterosexual men. Gay men who are less open about their sexual orientation and are less comfortable with being gay are more likely to experience anxiety during social interactions, which often means that social situations that are relatively innocuous for heterosexual men can be quite anxiety-provoking for some gay men.[55]

The findings are fairly consistent among members of the LGB community in that they often live under stressful circumstances and worry about negative evaluations and reactions from others. They also have realistic health concerns, which are often more critical for them than for heterosexuals; however, these individuals are more likely to take advantage of treatment.

RELIGIOUS GROUPS AND ANXIETY

Religious groups have also received attention in the research literature on Anxiety Disorders. Of course, religious beliefs themselves are not likely to be a risk factor, and even among people within the same religious group, beliefs can be fairly diverse. One study looked at a group of Christian and Jewish adults and found that religious denomination was a poor predictor of psychological distress, including anxiety and, in general, regardless of the specific religion, religiousness, religious practices, and positive religious core beliefs predicted lower levels of worry, lower trait anxiety, and lower depressive symptoms. Thus, one's religious background probably does not specifically influence one's development of psychological difficulties, but strongly held negative beliefs do predict increased psychological symptoms.[56] This implies that it is not the specific religious beliefs that are helpful or harmful but rather the possession of a spiritual belief system that does or does not provide comfort and answers to problems. Belonging to a spiritually involved community that provides validation for beliefs and nurturing when needed seems to offer a positive psychological perspective. This does not mean that in order to be mentally healthy one needs to join a religious group, but it does suggest that nurturing one's spirituality (not the same as religious devotion) and being a member of a spiritual community may provide opportunities to some people to give and receive support from others.

SUMMARY

Millions of Americans suffer from Anxiety Disorders, but only a small percentage of them receive the adequate treatment necessary to live a normal life. Billions of dollars are lost annually in productivity and disability, and minimal financial resources are focused on actual medical and psychological treatments. Countless relationships, families, friendships, jobs, careers, goals, and interests are disturbed or lost due to undiagnosed or undertreated Anxiety Disorders. Primary care physicians and mental health professionals must become cognizant of the variety of symptom patterns frequently presented by people of different sexes, ages, cultures, sexual orientations, and ethnicities. Early, accurate diagnoses and appropriate treatment or referrals to mental health professionals are essential to providing appropriate care.

Anxiety Disorders affect people worldwide; however, cultural norms often dictate the circumstances or events that lead to the development of symptoms and can determine whether the seeking of treatment is encouraged or even allowed. Some people or groups are more vulnerable to developing Anxiety Disorders, depending on the number of risk factors that affect them, access to needed treatment varies. Although recognizing the symptoms of Anxiety Disorders can be a challenge, it is clear from the research literature that combinations of medication and CBT are the most effective treatments. However, it is important for those who suffer from symptoms of persistent anxiety to seek treatment as soon as possible. Unfortunately for many, access to local, outpatient treatment locations depends on government or privately subsidized clinics and facilities, which often have a waiting period, or they are controlled by insurance companies that will only cover treatments deemed medically necessary and will rarely cover an inpatient hospital stay. Getting the right kinds of treatment is, unfortunately, a very difficult process for many, and this is a problem that will only get worse if we do not do a better job of meeting these needs.

4

Theories of Anxiety Disorders

The source of anxiety lies in the future. If you can keep the future out of mind, you can forget your worries.
                              —Milan Kundera, Czech novelist, playwright, and poet

Anxiety Disorders are complex and multifaceted experiences involving many physical and psychological symptoms. A number of theories offer a variety of explanations and causes, which at first may be confusing, but continuing extensive research has led to the development of new approaches, improved theories, and more effective treatments. While it may be tempting to consider which theory is the "correct" one, it is important to understand that no single theory can explain all of the phenomena—including biological, psychological, and cognitive factors—that are involved in an Anxiety Disorder. I encourage you to review each theory as a way to learn about this illness; in the final analysis, you will most likely answer the question, "What causes Anxiety Disorder?" with the reply, "All of the above."

BIOLOGICAL THEORIES

Anxiety and panic attacks look and feel to be biologically and possibly genetically based since most of the symptoms are physical in nature, and Anxiety Disorders tend to run in families. That a variety of medications are effective in treating anxiety seems to imply that the drug is fixing something at the biological level. But rigorous research in this area continues as we try to understand the mechanisms behind the biological factors involved in the development of an Anxiety Disorder. Some assert that genetic contributions play a significant role, while others have focused on structural issues in the brain. Others have examined the role of various neurotransmitters within the central nervous system, and most of the prescribed medical treatments that are effective in treating Anxiety Disorders work by modifying the way these neurotransmitter systems function.

For decades researchers have tried to unlock the genetic secrets in an effort to discover how genes may contribute to the development of Anxiety Disorders. Compelling evidence from a number of family studies demonstrates that people who have various specific types of Anxiety Disorders are more likely to be related to someone who suffers from the same disorder than those identified in the general public.[1] Other studies have shown that the presence of Anxiety Disorders in first- and second-degree relatives of Anxiety Disorder patients (immediate family and close relatives) is significantly high.[2] Fyer et al. found that Specific as well as Social Phobias tend to run in families, and, although the phobias usually involve various phobic objects, the frequency of phobias increases within families who have members who suffer from phobias.[3]

One of the challenges to understanding the role of genetics in anxiety disorders is that increased rates of psychological problems in family members of anxiety patients may be due to similar environments, observational learning, or other nonbiological psychological or social factors. For example, researchers will note the frequency of diagnosed psychopathology among family members, since it is often impossible to obtain specific diagnoses of relatives due to confidentiality issues. It is, therefore, difficult to determine whether other psychological problems within the family are anxiety based or due to the presence of another type of psychopathology that is causing an increase in anxiety conditions.

Another line of anxiety research in the genetic arena involves studies of sets of twins. One common criticism of these studies, however, is that twins tend to share an environment that is even more similar than their family members share, including non-twin siblings. Some twin studies have avoided this issue by studying twins who were raised together and twins who were raised separately due to a family situation that required them to be separated at birth or shortly thereafter. Most researchers have concluded that there is higher concordance for Anxiety Disorders in monozygotic (identical) twins than for dizygotic (fraternal) twins,[4] implying that, even for twins who share the same environment, those with an identical genetic makeup are more likely to share Anxiety Disorder than fraternal twins, who are no more alike genetically than other siblings. There is never a 100 percent concordance (all twin pairs having the same disorder) in studies examining identical twins, which strongly suggests that Anxiety Disorders cannot be due *only* to genetics or identical twins would each always have the same disorder.

One major study examined the genetic and environmental risk factors for Anxiety Disorders in men and women and did not report any gender differences for six different Anxiety Disorders.[5] However, two genetic factors were related to different types of Anxiety Disorders: one predisposed people to Generalized Anxiety Disorder (GAD), Panic Disorder (PD), and Agoraphobia and the other to Specific Phobias. They also found that people with Social Phobia seem to possess both types of genetic structures. It was also reported that an individual's experiences were key elements in the development of Social Phobia and Agoraphobia.

Many have concluded that there is also a genetic basis for Obsessive-Compulsive Disorder (OCD), and researchers at Johns Hopkins University have identified a promising genetic candidate that appears to be related to the early-onset type of OCD in which men seem to predominate.[6] Another interesting study found that OCD patients with one genotype responded to paroxetine (Paxil), those with a different genotype responded to venlafaxine XR (Effexor XR), and those who possessed both genotypes responded to either drug.[7] A genotype is just what it sounds like—the specific type of genetic profile for a person. Sharing a genotype does not mean that people with similar Anxiety Disorders share the same complete genetic structure, as in identical twins, but rather that they share a specific type of genetic structure related to a specific characteristic. The fact that patients who share a genotype are more likely to respond to the same medication suggests that a genetic component underlies the OCD.

Current research suggests that, rather than directly inheriting an Anxiety Disorder, people inherit the predisposition for developing one. We have known for some time that people can inherit a tendency to be tense or uptight[8] and that the contributions from several genes on different chromosomes collectively can make us vulnerable to anxiety when the critical psychological and social factors are in place.[9] This is an example of a diathesis-stress type of theory (as mentioned in chapter 3), which posits that an inherited predisposition to develop a certain problem (diathesis) is not manifested unless a specific environmental condition (stress) is also present.

Experiencing panic also tends to run in families, and this may have a genetic component as well.[10] Some evidence indicates that genetic contributions to panic and to anxiety differ,[11] but in both situations, genetic vulnerability, particularly in people under stress, may create a condition where panic might result, even if these factors do not cause the panic directly. In sum, the exact nature of the genetic link to anxiety is not yet fully understood, but it may be related to certain personality factors that are highly heritable (e.g., emotionality, introversion) rather than to the direct genetic transmission of anxiety itself.

Recent research has also examined the role of certain structures in the central nervous system and how they relate to the development of anxiety, with much of the work focusing on the amygdala, a structure in the brain's limbic system. The limbic system is sometimes called the pleasure center, but more appropriately it is related to the expression of emotions and is involved in coordinating different neurotransmitters that are implicated in the development and expression of an Anxiety Disorder.[12] There is a consensus among researchers and theorists about the crucial role of the amygdala, as well as the anterior cingulate cortex and the insula, in the pathophysiology of Anxiety Disorders. Advances in brain imaging techniques have helped our understanding of the involvement of certain brain structures and have validated some of the neurobiological hypotheses in Anxiety Disorders. Also, there is increasing speculation that some central nervous system structures may be the underlying causal factors involved in the etiology (cause) of some Anxiety Disorders.[13]

Some researchers have focused on the corticotrophin releasing factor, which stimulates the hypothalamic-pituitary-adrenal axis (HPA), causing a wide range of effects on the brain, including the limbic system. The HPA directly and indirectly affects a number of the neurotransmitter systems as well as the presence of fear, anxiety, and other emotional states. The limbic system is associated with anxiety[14] and acts as a mediator between the brain stem and the cerebral cortex. The more primitive brain stem monitors and senses changes in bodily functions and relays these potentially dangerous signals to higher cortical processes through the limbic system. Gray has identified a system in the brain that he calls the behavioral inhibition system (BIS), which is activated by signals from the brain stem when unexpected events, such as major changes in body functioning, might be an indication of danger.[15] When we see or directly sense danger, the signal is transmitted from the cortex to the septal-hippocampal system, where emotional changes will result. Whether the BIS is activated by signals that arise from the brain stem or descend from the cortex, our tendency is to freeze, experience anxiety, and apprehensively evaluate the situation to confirm that danger is present.[15] Gray and McNaughten suggest that the neural mechanisms in panic are different from those in anxiety and that they involve the fight-or-flight systems, resulting sometimes in panicky behavior; the researchers think this may be due to a deficiency in the serotonin system.[16]

As promising as some of the neuroimaging data have been, most of the recent research in the biological arena regarding Anxiety Disorders is in the area of neurotransmitters, which are the chemicals that carry messages from one neuron (brain cell) to another. The neurotransmitter systems most frequently associated with anxiety include gamma-aminobutyric acid (GABA), norepinephrine or noradrenalin (the noradrenergic system), serotonin (the serotonergic system), corticotrophic releasing factor, and dopamine (the dopaminergic system). However, the same systems may not be involved in each type of Anxiety Disorder. Evidence suggests that several neurotransmitters or neuromodulators such as serotonin, noradrenaline, adenosine, GABA, and cholecystokinin-4 all play a role in Panic Disorder,[17] implying that panic and anxiety are not qualitatively the same reactions either biologically or psychologically.

Serotonin has recently been at the forefront of anxiety research, partially because selective serotonin reuptake inhibitors have been successful in the treatment of a number of different Anxiety Disorders, including Phobias and Panic Disorder. Tancer et al. suggest an association between Social Phobia and selective supersensitivity in the serotonin system.[18] However, Social Phobia cannot simply be a serontonergic problem, because Schweizer et al. reported a relationship between dopamine and Social Phobia and found that Social Phobia tends to respond differently than Panic Disorder to various classes of medication.[19] Also, Kim et al.[20] have hypothesized that dysfunction within the serotonergic system plays an important role in Panic Disorder and not just in Social Phobias.

Although serotonin is important to the understanding and treatment of various Anxiety Disorders, many feel that anxiety is primarily mediated by the GABA-benzodiazepine system. Traditionally, benzodiazepine tranquilizers have been (and still are for some providers) the first line of treatment for Anxiety Disorders. Although these drugs are effective, they are not prescribed as much now as they have been in the past due to undesirable side effects such as cognitive slowing, decreased reaction time and coordination, and possible dependency. There is no question that the GABA system is related to anxiety and must be considered as part of the whole picture.

Considering all of the information regarding genetics, brain structures, and neurotransmitters, it is tempting to conclude that problems with anxiety are due to underlying biological factors and that the best way to treat Anxiety Disorders is through the use of medication or other medical treatments. However, a substantial amount of research supports alternative theories, and anxiety is not as simple as too much or too little of certain chemicals in the brain. Genetic factors may be involved in some, but not all, cases of Anxiety Disorder, and in cases certain brain systems or processes may be responsible. However, environmental changes can alter the levels of sensitivity in critical brain circuits, which can also lead to anxiety problems.[21] For example, cigarette smoking during adolescence is associated with a significantly increased risk for developing Anxiety Disorders, particularly GAD and PD, as an adult.[22] Whether this is due to brain changes associated with smoking or because these teens are more likely to be exposed to other environmental causes of anxiety while smoking is yet to be determined, but it certainly is an example of a behavior that leads to an increased susceptibility for developing Anxiety Disorders or that causes changes in the brain related to anxiety.

Many Anxiety Disorders are associated with self-reported symptoms of insomnia and fatigue, including GAD, PTSD, Social Phobia, and Panic Disorder, although only GAD and PTSD have specific sleep criteria in their diagnostic formulations. Sleep is one of the phenomena that is affected by both physiological and psychological factors, and people with Anxiety Disorders often suffer from insomnia (difficulty sleeping at night).[23] The psychological and physiological mechanisms related to Anxiety Disorders and insomnia are not fully understood, but it is such a common occurrence that most clinicians who work with patients with Anxiety Disorder find that they must also help them deal with sleep issues.

PSYCHOLOGICAL THEORIES

Psychodynamic Approaches

In addition to biological models, a number of psychological approaches are involved in understanding the development of Anxiety Disorders. The psychodynamic theorists typically look to a person's experiences in early life that are recorded in the subconscious mind as the primary causes of anxiety. Freud's theory, called psychoanalysis, dates back about a century and is certainly the most well known and influential psychodynamic theory.[24] Freud postulated that the human mind is composed of three basic psychological organs: the *id*, the instinctual basis of all human psychological energy; the *ego*, the adaptive organ of personality; and the *superego*, the internalization of morals and values acquired from the environment. Within the superego, there is the *superego ideal*, which represents the person one would like to become and the conscience, which provides internal guidance as to what is right and what is wrong. A child is born only with the id, considered the repository of all psychic energy; it originally derives from the biological energy system and then becomes independent. The id has two sources of energy: eros, the life energies, which largely involve libido or basic sexual energy—in Freud's system that does not just mean basic sexual desires but rather any type of experience that is fundamentally pleasurable—and thanatos, the death instinct, which is responsible for destructive and aggressive types of behaviors. Thus, the id is composed of these basic sexual and aggressive instincts and operates on the "primary process," which means that the id requires that its basic needs be fulfilled immediately and completely.

Realistically, it is impossible for all needs to be completely and immediately satisfied, so, as the id interacts with reality, a new organ emerges called the ego. The ego functions to fulfill the needs of the id within the constraints imposed by reality (society) and by the superego (conscience). It is the adaptive part of personality that is responsible for higher mental functioning (perception, cognition, learning) and operates on the "secondary process," which takes into account the constraints within which the ego must function. According to Freud, the ego must serve three harsh masters: the id, reality, and the superego. As the child develops, he begins to internalize the values and moral standards of society, largely as represented by the parents, and will develop the superego, which is responsible for people following the rules of society. If we do not follow the rules, we then feel guilty and remorseful.

Freud's theory of anxiety is based on the concept of being overwhelmed by those forces over which we feel we have no control. He suggests that the experience of birth is the prototype of all future anxiety. The unborn infant is living in a warm, moist, pleasant environment where she does not even have to eat—there is minimal stimulation, and most of it is pleasurable. During birth these comfortable conditions are significantly disrupted; after being squeezed and forced through the birth canal, the baby is often thrust into a bright, noisy, and possibly painful environment, where it first experiences hunger pains and has to actually eat. For Freud, this was the most vivid example of overstimulation and provides the basis upon which people try to minimize or at least to control the levels of stimulation throughout the rest of their lives. This fear of overstimulation is the basis of all anxiety, according to Freud. He postulated three basic types of anxiety: *Reality anxiety*, which we call fear, is based on a realistic threat in the environment that the ego first assesses and then concludes that there is a realistic possibility of environmental factors overwhelming us with undesirable stimuli. For example, if we are walking through the woods and see a bear running toward us, we will experience the fear (reality anxiety) of overstimulation (being mauled or bitten) by the bear. *Neurotic anxiety* is based on a conflict between the ego and the id; the fear of the ego being overwhelmed by id impulses. If the id has sexual or aggressive impulses that it wants fulfilled, but the ego assesses the environment (reality) and concludes that this fulfillment is inappropriate, it will create the fear of what might happen if these unacceptable impulses were allowed expression, and this is called neurotic anxiety. Freud also postulated *moral anxiety*, the fear that is produced when a person does, thinks, or imagines something that violates the standards of the superego, and this is generally referred to as *guilt*. According to Freud, anxiety is a signal to the ego of impending overstimulation by realistic fears, unacceptable id impulses, or by thoughts and behaviors that may lead to trouble by violating the rules of the superego. Children struggle with fears and feelings about controlling their environment, and it is the actions of parents during early childhood that seem to foster a sense of control or uncontrollability.[25]

Most of Freud's writings about neuroses address how people develop Anxiety Disorders, how they deal with it, and how it can be treated. Freud uses the word *neurosis* to refer to Anxiety Disorders, but he also included what we today call Somatoform and Dissociative Disorders, to be discussed later in chapters 10 and 11. Following Freud, other psychodynamic theorists have focused more on cognitive processes and less on the instinctual basis of anxiety. They, too, have looked to childhood experiences as the primary source of intrapsychic conflict that results in anxiety-related problems, but they more often consider the adult experiences and problems that result from the basic underlying causes of the anxiety.

Humanistic and Existential Approaches

The humanistic and existential theorists have developed different ideas about the origin of anxiety. Although they are somewhat similar to the psychodynamic theorists and focus on what is inside a person's mind, they are less concerned about the unconscious basis of personality functioning and focus more on the conscious mind and more immediate conflicts and problems. The humanistic theorists were mostly in vogue during the 1960s and 1970s, although philosophers and social theorists had written about humanistic approaches to understanding human behavior prior to that time. Carl Rogers and Abraham Maslow were influential theorists and practitioners who attracted many to their particular points of view. Both were elected to the presidency of the American Psychological Association, which is an indication of the support they had among psychologists and the lay public as well—especially students who were seeking unique ideas and different approaches to understanding people.

The humanistic approach deviates from the strictly deterministic and the more historically prominent theoretical models—the psychodynamic and behavioral theories. The humanists assert that humans are more than a composite of intrapsychic impulses or learned behaviors and that by only digging into an individual's psychic history to discover the unconscious instincts that might be producing conflicts completely misses the humanity and richness of the human experience that defines the individual. Similarly, they believe that the behavioral theory, which asserts that all behavior is caused by learning through interaction with the environment, is misguided as well. If a strictly deterministic approach to human behavior is followed, as with psychodynamic and behavioral theorists, then human factors, such as choice and free will, do not fit. The humanists feel strongly that trying to understand behavior by reducing it to simple instincts and learned behaviors does not do justice to the complexity of the human experience, thoughts, feelings, and actions.

Rogers's model of anxiety, the most well-developed and influential humanistic theory from the past, states that the *Self* is the fundamental structure of personality and the core of who we are and who we will become as a person.[26] He postulated that we all possess an inner mechanism called the *innate valuing tendency*, the basis upon which we judge and evaluate our experiences. Experiences that are consistent with the Self are viewed as good and healthy, while experiences that are inconsistent with the Self are considered bad or uncomfortable.

The difficulty that results from Rogers's theory is that, while we all have the need to seek out experiences that are consistent with our true selves, we also posses the *need for positive regard*, which is the need to feel good about ourselves as well as to have others feel good about us. Thus, we do things that will increase experiences that are consistent with our Self, but we also do things that we think will make other people value us. The resulting conflict between wanting to stay consistent with our Self and wanting to meet the expectations of others, results in our developing what is called *conditions of worth*. When the difference between the Self and our experiences grows, the inconsistency produces feelings of anxiety, which is also a signal (as in Freud's theory) that there is a discrepancy between our Self and our experience, and the Self may become disorganized, or even detached from reality. This potential threat is distinctly troubling, and the person may not even be aware of its origin.

Similar in many ways to the humanistic theories, the existential approach was popular a few decades ago. During the period between World War I and World War II, several European psychiatrists became dissatisfied with traditional psychoanalysis and began to consider existentialism, a branch of philosophy that included a new model for understanding human personality and experience. They drew from the existential philosophers Nietzsche, Heidegger, Kierkegaard, and Camus, plus a number of influential psychologists and psychiatrists, including Victor Frankl, who wrote about his experiences in a Nazi concentration camp during World War II; U.S. psychologist Rollo May; and Scottish psychiatrist R. D. Laing.

The existential theorists share many ideas with the humanists, although they tend to place more emphasis on the importance of choice and responsibility as well as the vital necessity of free will as fundamental to understanding the human condition. They are concerned with people making choices and decisions in their best interests and being true to themselves. They believe that the basis of anxiety is inauthenticity, which simply means not being true to oneself and exhibiting behavior that is not consistent with what is best and healthiest for oneself. However, as similar as their ideas seem to the humanistic theories, they have very different notions about psychopathology (abnormal psychology). Instead of regarding anxiety as an illness, they consider it an experience that results from the choices one makes throughout life and that one of those choices is to continue feeling anxious.

Behavioral Approaches

The behavioral and cognitive theorists produce a very different approach to understanding anxiety. While the behavioral theories have held a prominent position in the psychological models of psychopathology for about a century, some of the newer cognitive and cognitive-behavioral models are more inclusive of a broader variety of psychological factors and are not as narrow and restrictive as the earlier behavioral models. The earliest works of the behaviorists dealing with the development of anxiety dates back to Watson and Rayner.[27] In 1920 they demonstrated that a learned fear reaction could be taught to a youngster, "Little Albert," by using conditioning procedures. As an 18-month-old toddler, Albert was exposed to a white rat, which did not bother or concern him much. Then, while in the presence of the white rat, Watson made a loud noise, which startled Albert and made him cry. From that moment forward, Albert was frightened of the white rat. Thus, Watson and Rayner reported that a phobia could be acquired through conditioning. Today, of course, this type of study would be considered unethical and would not be permitted. However, during Watson's era, there were no rules or limitations, and, although some were very upset and concerned about his research methods, he had not violated any laws or standards of the time. From this somewhat questionable beginning, many researchers and theorists have pursued the idea that abnormal behavior, just as normal behavior, can be acquired through learning and conditioning and can be treated using the same types of learning approaches.

Rachman proposed three well-supported pathways to the acquisition of anxiety through condition/learning processes: classical conditioning, vicarious learning, and transmission via information or instructions.[28] Classical conditioning is the type of process that was responsible for Little Albert's acquired fear of rats. This approach to learning was first demonstrated in a laboratory by a Russian physiologist named Ivan Pavlov, who was studying digestion in dogs. While looking at the role of salivation in digestion, he found that he could place meat paste (unconditioned stimulus) on the dog's tongue and the dog would salivate (unconditioned response). Actually, Pavlov called the dog's reaction a reflex, but today psychologists refer to it as a response. He also noticed that after the dogs became aware of him in the laboratory they would begin to salivate the instant he walked into the room. However, Pavlov could not explain how this new response could occur in the absence of a direct stimulus. He then paired the meat paste (unconditioned stimulus) with a neutral stimulus—a bell, in this case (conditioned stimulus)—and the dog still salivated (unconditioned response, since the meat paste was still being used). Later, he discovered that when he rang the bell (conditioned stimulus), a new response would occur—salivating in response to the bell (conditioned response). This then became a new model of learning.

Watson and others tried to assert that classical conditioning could account for the development of different psychological disorders, but it was clear that this model was too limited. Based primarily on the research of behavioral psychologist B. F. Skinner, a new model of learning emerged: operant conditioning. With this approach no evoking stimulus is required; it is based on the idea that behavior can be shaped by its consequences. Like the earlier work of psychologist Edwin Thorndike, Skinner looked at what followed a given behavior and how it affected subsequent responses. The fundamental concept in operant conditioning is that reinforcement—what happens following a response—increases the probability that the response will occur again. Positive reinforcement means that a response is more likely to occur when a positive outcome is introduced following a specific behavior. This is much like a reward—if you want someone to continue doing something, you give them something positive. Further, negative reinforcement involves the removal of an aversive or negative outcome, and this too reinforces behavior. For example, I could reinforce a particular behavior in a laboratory rat by giving it a food pellet for responding correctly (positive reinforcement), or I could turn off a painful shock when it responded correctly (negative reinforcement). In both cases I have increased the probability of the correct response occurring again. Likewise, by removing the positive reinforcer (or not removing a negative reinforcer) you can discourage unwanted behavior, and it will cease in the absence of a reinforcer (extinction); or by adding a negative outcome or removing a positive one, you can directly punish the response. As it turns out, punishment is not usually as reliable as reward for changing behavior, but reinforcement or extinction is more effective. This does not mean that punishment can never be used to change behavior but that the use of reinforcement or extinction, when possible, is more efficient and more effective. Although some question the validity of this statement, decades of research support it.

Considering all of the concepts and theories of learning, as well as the techniques from both classical and operant conditioning, many theorists and researchers felt empowered with an arsenal of learning models to help them explain how Anxiety Disorders are acquired and reinforced. O. H. Mowrer developed the Two-Factor Theory, which became the basis for many therapeutic techniques used today.[29] Mowrer felt that classical conditioning could explain how learned fear reactions are acquired when people respond to a stimulus that is paired with a fearful event. Just like Little Albert, people can learn to be fearful in the presence of a stimulus that is not truly dangerous and that has not frightened them in the past. However, his theory did not explain why the fear persists over time. He showed how people become anxious while in the presence of the feared object and how the feelings of experienced anxiety are distinctly unpleasant. Thus, when a person withdraws from the feared stimulus, thereby reducing his anxiety, the person feels better and the avoidance behavior is reinforced. The removal of an aversive stimulus to reward a certain behavior is negative reinforcement, and this explains why a phobia or learned fear can persist even though the feared outcome never occurs. According to Mowrer, a phobia is learned by classical conditioning and is maintained by the avoidance of the phobic object. The control or reduction of anxiety negatively reinforces the avoidance behavior and is, therefore, perpetuated by operant conditioning. A significant problem when dealing with phobias is *generalization*, a process of fearful responses to additional stimuli or conditions, which may only be moderately similar to the originally feared stimulus. This is how phobias tend to increase over time.

As compelling as the behavioral theories are, they are not without their critics; nor is there one simple explanation as to why conditioning seems to work differently with some people. Not all cases of phobia show evidence of direct conditioning, and, even under conditions that seem as though they should lead to a learned fear reaction, not all people will develop a phobia.[30] In addition, learning methods other than conditioning can explain the origin of some learned anxiety reactions.[31] Finally, some theorists have stated that the conditioning theories do not explain the unequal distribution of learned fears within the general population.[32]

Behavioral theorist Albert Bandura's research demonstrates convincingly that during observational learning people can acquire complex behaviors by simply observing another person's behavior (modeling) or by watching another person learn and noting the consequences of that behavior (vicarious learning).[31] Observational learning appears to occur cognitively and does not require the person to perform the behavior themselves in order to learn, and it helps to explain the acquisition of complex behavior, including certain types of anxiety responses. Although this theory is grounded in the operant conditioning heritage, it was one of the first modern theories to incorporate cognitive factors into a learning model, and this set the stage for the newer cognitive and cognitive behavioral models that were to follow.

Although influential, the conditioning methods are not adequate to explain the variety of acquired fears or the reasons that some stimuli are more likely to lead to phobic reactions than others. Rachman suggests that there are biological factors that determine why some fears form and others do not.[28] Poulton and Menzies posit that some fears are not learned through associative pathways like conditioning but have evolutionary value and are, therefore, embedded within a person in a manner that is more likely to develop fears to certain types of things (e.g., snakes, spiders, heights, etc.).[33]

Seligman has put forward the concept of *preparedness* to explain why there is an unequal distribution of certain fears, favoring the hypothesis of an evolutionary tendency to fear certain stimuli for the protection of the species.[34] He suggests that preparedness accounts for the rapid and easy acquisition of some learned fear reactions. For example, it is easier to learn to fear snakes and spiders than it is to learn to fear a piece of chalk or a pencil. Seligman asserts that preparedness explains the irrationality behind some fears, how certain connections between stimuli and responses are more easily established, and why some learned fears are more resistant to extinction than others.

Other researchers have found that some people are more prone to develop fear reactions to some stimuli and that selective exposure to specific types of experiences during development is more likely to lead to an increase of phobias. Kagan et al. reported that, even as early as 18 months, the manner in which children interact with other individuals, toys, and objects tends to differ.[35] Behavior exhibited by the shy and withdrawn children is called *behavior inhibition* and may be a predisposing factor in the later development of Social Phobia and other Anxiety Disorders. Other findings from Bruch and Heimberg established that, when compared to nonanxious individuals, people with Social Phobia remember their parents discouraging them from socializing, placing undue importance on the opinions of others, and using shame as a means of discipline.[36] They also stated other predictors of Social Phobia, such as a childhood history of separation anxiety and self-consciousness or shyness and noted that these youngsters reported more shyness and a lower frequency of dating during adolescence.[36] Another factor in the development of Social Phobia is *perfectionism*, because the fear of making mistakes especially in the presence of others, is a major issue with this disorder.[37]

Cognitive Approaches

Conditioning and learning are important to understanding Anxiety Disorders, but they are not adequate explanations for the full range of factors related to anxiety. A more recent approach comes from the cognitive theorists that focuses upon attention, perception, and thinking, and how these processes affect the development and/or maintenance of anxiety. George Kelly, in the 1950s and 1960s, was one of the first to take the cognitive perspective further into the understanding of how cognitive processes are relevant to human personality and psychopathology.[38] His approach is called Personal Construct Theory, and it studies the ways in which people think about and anticipate events in their life. He felt that people use *constructs* to understand and anticipate the world—that is, to make sense of it. These constructs are cognitive structures that help us to organize information and ideas into coherent wholes that allow us to think and anticipate efficiently. Kelly's work was seminal and influenced many others, but it was not applied to clinical problems as early as other approaches.

Albert Ellis was one of the first psychologists to effectively build an entire approach to psychotherapy based upon cognitive techniques, and his ideas were quickly incorporated into therapeutic methods and training.[39] His approach, Rational-Emotive Psychotherapy, was influential during the 1960s and 1970s and there are still therapists who use his approach, although few identify themselves primarily as rational-emotive therapists. Ellis's ideas have significantly influenced the manner in which therapists work today and have helped to identify some of the dysfunctional ways people think about things and how to confront and change their thinking patterns.

More recently Beck and Emery began applying some new cognitive approaches to the understanding and treatment of anxiety.[40] Originally, Aaron Beck applied his cognitive approach to Depression, which has been a helpful and positive contribution to the understanding and treatment of this disorder. Then shifting their ideas and approaches to Anxiety Disorders, Beck and Emery applied some of Kelly's ideas about the development of constructs (ways of organizing information) to the development of anxiety. These constructs relate to the concepts of danger and vulnerability and to the person's estimation of her ability to cope with the danger.

Another recent cognitive model of anxiety is the fear of fear approach. Goldstein and Chambless suggest that following a panic attack people may learn to fear that any change in their physical state might indicate the possibility of another panic attack.[41] Thus, even low-level physical sensations become a conditioned stimulus that triggers fear and worry. Some researchers have pointed out that the fear of anxiety itself arises from the association of internal cues with panic attacks.[41] Although this model relies on cognitive factors, it also employs physiological and behavioral elements. However, the fear of fear concept is the central notion and depends upon beliefs about anxiety, danger, and vulnerability. The cognitive portion relates to the ways people think about minor physical changes or about the risks they fear, which are present in response to the *possibility* that they might experience feelings of anxiety. This often results in an overreaction to minor physical changes and a mental exaggeration of the dangers and risks associated with anxiety.

Reiss and McNally developed a similar model called the Anxiety Sensitivity Model, which is based on the notion that some people believe that experiencing anxiety can cause illness, embarrassment, or additional anxiety and leads to more significant problems.[42] While this is an extension of the fear of fear model, it rests on the assumption that the belief structure is the fundamental reason why anxiety becomes more intense and problematic for some people.

Most of the cognitive models of Anxiety Disorders have emphasized the role of *selective information processing*, and research has shown that this bias can occur very quickly and with very little information. When Anxiety Disorders develop, due in part to attentional biases, it is an indication that treatment should focus on the biases or dysfunctional ways of thinking. In fact, one treatment approach called cognitive bias modification is a promising way of dealing with attentional bias in the development of emotional problems such as Anxiety Disorders.[43]

Literature suggests that patients with Anxiety Disorders are characterized by an attentional bias for threatening information and toward frightening interpretations of ambiguous information. It also reports that a memory bias favoring recall of threatening information occurs in Panic Disorder but rarely in other types of Anxiety Disorders. The bias of increased attention toward stimuli that suggest a threat or danger is very common among anxiety patients, and treatments that focus on these biases have been promising.[44]

Some research has found that attentional bias toward negative social cues can serve an etiological (causal) and/or maintenance role in Social Anxiety Disorder[45] and that by using attention training techniques patients can be taught to focus less of their attention on cues that suggest danger or vulnerability. This training was effective in reducing both Social and Trait Anxiety, and the treatment gains were still present four months following the end of therapy. Other researchers report that people with either Social or Specific Phobias devote more attention to threat-related information than do non-phobic patients.[46] As mentioned above, perfectionism as a personality trait is also related to Social Phobia, because the fear of making mistakes is of primary concern of people with this disorder.[37] Thus, if people believe that they cannot make a mistake without experiencing catastrophic consequences and that they must never make a mistake, it is easy to understand how perfectionism can be related to Social Anxiety.

A similar issue for anxiety patients is the predictability of stimuli. It is assumed that when aversive stimuli are less predictable, they will be more anxiety provoking. However, the research literature demonstrates that anxiety levels are quite comparable regardless of how predictable the aversive stimuli are but that patients prefer predictability regardless of the anxiety level.[47]

Another line of research in the cognitive realm demonstrates that older patients with anxiety problems have difficulty with cognitive processing. For example, speed of cognitive processing, the ability to shift attention, and cognitive inhibition are frequently less efficient in the anxious elderly patient. Although many elderly patients suffer from depression *and* anxiety, this research found that depressive symptoms alone were not associated with any cognitive deficits.[48] Therefore, at least in older adults, anxiety does appear to interfere with cognitive functioning.

Although the cognitive approaches have been beneficial in the development of theories and treatments for Anxiety Disorders, they have limitations as well. Theorists refer to cognitive predispositions for dealing with certain types of information in specific ways called *schemata* (singular is a *schema*). These cognitive templates, through which information is channeled and processed, might function to elicit anxiety responses in some people. However, if the cognitive schemata are the triggering mechanisms for anxiety, where do the schemata come from? Since they must be either acquired or inherent, they are either learned by the person through experiences or are part of the biological system and hard-wired into the brain. In either case, this aspect of the cognitive model depends upon another and different type of model (learning or biological) to explain why cognitions lead to anxiety.

In addition to questions about the origins of schemata and one's predisposition to develop anxiety problems, there are concerns about one's level of vulnerability. If people acquire a potentially troublesome cognitive schema, why are some people more likely to have this schema? And even for those who share a schema, why are some people more likely to develop anxiety than others? There must be something in the person's makeup that determines whether anxiety will emerge from certain cognitive predispositions.

The conclusion that can be drawn from these findings is that cognitive factors are an important contribution to the understanding and treatment of Anxiety Disorders. However, it is obvious that cognitive factors alone do not explain everything about the causes of anxiety and that, as helpful as they are, we must rely on other factors to make sense of the complex world of anxiety.

INTEGRATING THE DIFFERENT THEORIES

To fully understand and appreciate Anxiety Disorders, emerging data from the research, theory, and treatment areas suggest that it is necessary to combine ideas and approaches from the different models and theories. Gorman et al. point out the remarkable similarity between the physiological and behavioral consequences of panic attacks in humans and conditioned fear responses in animals.[49] These include autonomic arousal, fear evoked by specific situations, and avoidance of these cues. The researchers hypothesize that there is a fear network of systems in the brain and that activation of this network produces biological and behavioral reactions similar to those associated with panic attacks. The researchers go on to suggest the presence of a similar network in humans that is associated with panic attacks. Further, Lonsdorf et al. note that, while classical conditioning can explain the acquisition and extinction of fear responses, there are different systems within the brain that are also associated with acquisition and extinction.[50] This, too, suggests that we must rely on both the psychological and biological realms of understanding to fully explain these concepts.

Although fear and anxiety are similar and related, they are mediated by different brain systems. Experiencing anxiety seems to lower the threshold for fear, which means that if you are anxious you are more likely to become fearful as well. However, since anxiety and fear are not always realistic and can occur in the absence of a real threat—or at least be disproportionate to a threat—there must be something else occurring. For example, it appears that cognitive appraisal of threat is an important element to understand how fear and anxiety occur. If a person is feeling fearful or anxious, the experience, in part, may be influenced or moderated by how he perceive and/or thinks about what is happening to him.

With every new study, the emerging model of anxiety becomes more complex, and many favor an integrated model as discussed by Barlow.[10] Most psychological accounts of panic invoke conditioning and cognitive explanations that are difficult to separate.[51] Further, stressful life events can trigger biological and psychological vulnerabilities to anxiety, and the expression of that anxiety involves both psychological and biological mechanisms. The integrative models combine the biological, behavioral, psychological, social, and other related factors in an effort to explain the causes and manifestations of anxiety and are becoming part of accepted treatments.

WHO IS VULNERABLE?

One line of inquiry has examined issues of patient vulnerability, focusing on various factors that make people more susceptible to Anxiety Disorders and on how to prevent, minimize, and treat them. This includes an examination of the diathesis part of the diathesis-stress model for these disorders, which means trying to understand any conditions or characteristics that might predispose a person to develop an Anxiety Disorder.

Some predisposing factors may be biological, and in primate studies, Suomi documented substantial individual differences in the degree and intensity of anxiety-like behaviors in infant and juvenile rhesus monkeys.[52] Additional research found several factors related to behavioral inhibition in human children that emerge very early and are consistent through childhood and adolescence. These behaviors include clinging to the mother, crying easily, and a reluctance to interact with others—behaviors that are much like anxiety.[53] One difficulty is that children often cannot identify the emotions they are experiencing, and, even after looking at anxiety-provoking stimulus pictures, some children still did not identify themselves as being anxious, although they showed higher levels of somatic arousal.[54] Psychological traits (e.g., introversion, activity level, startle response, etc.) also may relate to the later development of anxiety, and these, too, are stable throughout childhood and adolescence.

Additional physical factors that can affect someone's vulnerability for developing Anxiety Disorder have been explored, and some researchers suggest a relationship between Panic Disorder and a cardiac condition called mitral valve prolapse,[55] but this hypothesis has yielded inconsistent and inconclusive results. Other research shows that post-myocardial infarction (heart attack) patients who experience in-hospital complications following their heart attack have higher levels of anxiety that appear to be independent of any Depression they might experience.[56] Another physical factor implicated in Panic Disorder and Agoraphobia (fear of being in unfamiliar or fearful situations) is the vestibular system, which is related to the sense of balance in the inner ear. People suffering from anxiety often complain of feeling dizzy or light-headed, and people with Panic Disorder tend to overinterpret physical symptoms, focus on them, and amplify their impact. Further, people with Agoraphobia usually suffer from Panic Disorder, so it is apparent how these two disorders are possibly related to vestibular difficulties or might at least be influenced by these physical factors.

Sleep is another factor that affects one's vulnerability to developing Anxiety Disorders. Chorney et al. found that in primary care settings about 10 percent to 30 percent of children experience sleep disturbances, whereas in community mental health centers (37%) and child clinics (47%) even more children present with sleep problems. One longitudinal (over time) study found that early childhood sleep problems were associated with Anxiety Disorders 20 years later; some of the sleep problems included difficulty falling or staying asleep, nightmares, insomnia, and abrupt awakening.[57]

A model developed at the Cornell Panic-Anxiety Study Group has led to interesting findings regarding vulnerability factors for Anxiety Disorders and to the development of some treatment approaches.[58] Researchers discovered that people at risk for Panic Disorder have a neurophysiological vulnerability to experience panic attacks and/or multiple developmental traumas. The child becomes frightened of unfamiliar situations and becomes excessively dependent on the primary caregiver to protect them. The child can develop psychological predispositions to panic and anxiety as a result of these fears and conflicts. Others have demonstrated that childhood trauma appears to have particularly powerful and long-lasting effects and that, after controlling for other factors, childhood trauma has been associated with the development of many psychiatric disorders, including Anxiety and Dissociative Disorders.[59]

One situation that can cause a parent or family member to be more vulnerable to one of the types of Anxiety Disorders known as Posttraumatic Stress Disorder is having a child with a chronic illness. Few events in life are as traumatic as having a child develop a serious and chronic medical condition, especially if the disease is potentially fatal. Within the general population, the incidence of PTSD is 1.3 percent to 9.2 percent, depending on the study. However, in parents with a seriously and chronically ill child, the rate for mothers developing PTSD is 19.6 percent, for fathers it is 11.6 percent, and for all parents it is 22.8 percent.[60] It is important to be aware of PTSD symptoms in caregiving parents (which is discussed in detail in chapter 6), to adequately treat the symptoms so the parents can be the most effective caregivers possible, and to prevent a more serious problem from developing later.

SUMMARY

Many factors are involved in the causes of Anxiety Disorders, ranging from biological and psychological to social and cultural. No simple model of anxiety exists, but recent studies and theories have improve the understanding and treatment of Anxiety Disorders. With continuing research comes new and improved treatments, and we know that when people with Anxiety Disorders receive adequate treatment, they typically improve.

5

Physical Responses and Types of Anxiety Disorders I: Generalized Anxiety Disorder and Panic Disorder

> When I came to Hollywood, I could wear a bikini, but I was in misery because people were looking at me. So I wore baggy clothes and watched other girls get the big parts and awards. I used to go home and play piano and scream at night to let out my frustrations. And this led to my agoraphobia.
> —Kim Basinger, American actor

To understand the various types of Anxiety Disorders and the differences between them, it is important to know how anxiety and stress impact us physically and psychologically. Although there are several different types of Anxiety Disorders, anxiety is the fundamental basis of each of them. Anxiety and stress are often correlated, and the physical responses to stress look and feel very much like anxiety. Further, stress can lead to feelings of anxiety and anxiety can be a source of stress, and in some disorders anxiety may only be secondary to the primary problem.

PHYSICAL RESPONSES TO STRESS AND ANXIETY

Responses of the Brain

When we experience acute stress (e.g., being chased by a bear in the woods), the brain responds in several ways. The hypothalamic-pituitary-adrenal axis (HPA) is activated and immediately affects different processes in the body. The brain structure called the hypothalamus (part of the limbic system) is connected to the pituitary gland and the adrenal glands, which are also involved in how the body reacts to stress. After the HPA is activated, the release of steroid hormones and the stress hormone called cortisol activate the fight-or-flight system by arousing the body to take decisive action to reduce the threat—either aggress (fight) or escape (flight). Clearly, this system predates our human ancestors and is of distinct evolutionary value for the protection of the species.

As the stress continues or worsens, the release of catecholamines and the activation of the amygdala (sometimes called the fear center) occur. The amygdala is a small structure deep in the brain that controls major emotional activities such as fear and anxiety in addition to depression, aggression, and affection. Catecholamines are chemicals (like adrenalin) that activate the sympathetic branch of the autonomic nervous system, which deals with those systems related to the fight-or-flight responses (e.g., blood pressure, heart rate, breathing rate). The catecholamines also suppress activity in the frontal lobes, which are concerned with short-term memory, concentration, inhibition, and rational thought. Therefore, the autonomic nervous system allows us to act quickly in an emergency without thinking, but it also interferes with the processing of complex information or tasks. Simultaneously, the neurotransmitters signal the hippocampus (another area in the brain) to store the emotionally loaded experience into the long-term memory area, which then allows us to learn from difficult or frightening experiences.

Responses by the Heart, Lungs, and Circulatory System

When the brain processes threat information, the heart rate and blood pressure increase almost instantly. The breathing rate also climbs, allowing the lungs to increase their oxygen intake. The spleen discharges more red and white blood cells, making it possible for the blood to carry more oxygen throughout the body, and the blood flow can increase 300–400 percent, priming the muscles, lungs, and brain to handle more demands under stressful or dangerous conditions.

Responses by the Immune System

When a person is experiencing acute anxiety or stress, the immune system is also affected. Steroid types of hormones dampen parts of the immune system, causing specific infection fighters or other immune molecules to redistribute to where injury or infection is occurring (e.g., the skin, bone marrow, and lymph nodes). Acute stress can help the immune system in some cases, but just in the short term. When stress is long lasting or intense, it will interfere with normal immune system functioning. It is not imaginary that people tend to become ill more easily or heal more slowly when they are experiencing stress.

Responses in the Mouth and Throat

When we are stressed, fluids are diverted from nonessential locations, including the mouth and throat, to other parts of the body. You may have noticed that when stressed or anxious, your mouth and throat become dry or you may experience muscle spasms in the throat, making it difficult to talk and swallow. Although this is not dangerous, it can be frightening to someone who does not understand what is happening. This explains why people with Anxiety Disorders, who frequently experience dry mouth, often fear that their throat is closing up and that they will suffocate.

Skin Responses

During a stressful or anxious time, blood is diverted from the skin to more essential functions, which helps to reduce blood loss from injury and may result in a cool and clammy feeling. The scalp also tightens so that the hair feels as though it is standing straight up. The phrases, "It would make your skin crawl" and "That would make the hair stand up on the back of your neck," refer to the skin's response to fear, stress, or anxiety.

Metabolic Responses

When the body is preparing for fight or flight, blood is diverted to the brain and skeletal muscles so that quick action can occur; at the same time, the digestive system shuts or slows down for a short time. It is not uncommon for people who are attuned to physical changes to interpret these digestive system changes as clinically significant and worrisome.

Physical Responses When Stress or Anxiety Disappears or When It Continues

As the external stressor disappears, the stress hormones return to normal levels and the body's systems return to normal functioning. However, if stress is continuous, if multiple stressors are present, if the person is acutely anxious, or if the resulting arousal is not soon alleviated, systemic problems can result in the development of disease-like states. When an organ system is overloaded for a long period, its ability to function normally can be significantly impaired. The systems most likely to react are those that have been previously weakened by disease or other problems or are the most normally reactive and, thus, predisposed to developing problems. Everyone has one (or a few) systems that are the most likely to respond to stress, such as headaches, high blood pressure, and upset stomach. These systems are homeostatic, meaning that they automatically seek to return to normal levels when over- or understimulated, but if stress and anxiety are significant or continuing, the body may overcorrect and develop further problems. For example, if a person's digestive system has slowed under stress, but the stress or anxiety is intense or continues, the body tries to reset at the homeostatic level but may overcorrect, resulting in an upset stomach or digestive problems such as diarrhea. For a detailed explanation of how bodily systems are affected by stress and anxiety, consider visiting a website created at the University of Maryland[1] and listed in the back of this book in the Resources section.

Other Sources of Anxiety-like Symptoms

A number of medical conditions can produce symptoms that are similar to those seen with anxiety or with acute anxiety attacks. For example, people who are withdrawing from heavy alcohol or drug use will often experience severe anxiety-like symptoms. If a careful history reveals that anxiety problems did not exist prior to the alcohol or drug abuse, then the symptoms are clearly the result of withdrawal. If the anxiety was present before the substance abuse, then the Anxiety Disorder preexisted and must be treated along with the dependence. Even medical conditions such as asthma and heart attacks can produce anxiety, which is understandable given what the body experiences during such medical crises. Another medical condition that can produce anxiety-like symptoms is hyperthyroidism. The prefix *hyper* means too much of something. Therefore, hyperthyroidism means that the thyroid is producing too much of the thyroid hormones, and it will create an overarousal that feels and looks like anxiety. Similarly, a deficiency in folate or vitamin B$_{12}$ can produce symptoms similar to anxiety. Women going through menopause frequently notice an increase in general anxiety and worrying and, while this may be transitory, it is still troublesome and usually responds well to treatment. Finally, other medical problems such as gastrointestinal disease and some infectious diseases can produce anxiety or anxiety-like symptoms.

Some medications can produce side effects similar to anxiety. Bronchodilators such as ephedrine or epinephrine that treat breathing problems can also cause anxiety types of symptoms. Psychostimulants such as methylphenidate (Ritalin) or related drugs such as amphetamines, can also produce symptoms similar to anxiety, as can taking too high a dose of thyroid hormone.

Chronic anxiety can cause significant and disturbing physical symptoms that interfere with one's life and happiness. Over time, severe anxiety can increase the risk of hypertension and heart attack, although anxiety may not be the direct cause these conditions. Left untreated, chronic anxiety can produce a higher risk for other medical and psychological conditions.

TYPES OF ANXIETY DISORDERS I

Each type of Anxiety Disorders has its own distinctive symptoms, problems, and specific types of treatments. It is also common for Anxiety Disorders to have comorbid conditions (physical or psychological conditions that are co-existing), which can frequently confuse the diagnostic picture. But first it is important to understand the major types of Anxiety Disorders, their unique symptoms, and how they differ, beginning with two of the more common: Generalized Anxiety Disorder and Panic Disorder.

Generalized Anxiety Disorder

Generalized Anxiety Disorder (GAD) is characterized by pervasive and continuous feelings of anxiety and/or excessive worrying. Because it is frequently a comorbid condition, some professionals have questioned whether it is an independent disorder or whether it always exists as part of another disorder. Patients are sometimes not diagnosed with GAD because the symptoms are not recognized as a separate problem. Even the research literature has not focused much on GAD due to shifting diagnostic criteria, the relatively low diagnostic reliability, and questions about the diagnostic validity of the disorder.[2] However, most professionals still consider GAD an acceptable diagnostic category, and in recent years inroads have been made into further understanding and improving treatment options.

About 1.6 percent of the general population suffers from GAD, with a 12-month prevalence of 3.1 percent. This means that, during any 12-month period, about 3 percent of the population will be diagnosed with GAD. The lifetime prevalence rate is 5.1 percent, which means that, over the span of a life, over 5 percent of people will suffer from GAD at some point. Although a relatively high percentage of people experience this common disorder, it does not receive as much attention as Panic Disorder. Interestingly, GAD is commonly diagnosed and treated in primary care settings but is one of the least common disorders followed in mental health centers,[2] implying that people who suffer from GAD are either not referred to mental health professionals, or when they are, another condition is diagnosed as the primary issue.

Twenty-two percent of primary care patients complain of anxiety problems, a rate much higher than in the general population and in mental health settings. While GAD is found more in women and in middle-aged and older patients, it is less frequently diagnosed in adolescents and younger adults. GAD results in a significant number of disability days (similar to Depression) and is often comorbid with Depression, making the disability burden even higher. Appropriate diagnosis and use of psychological and medical treatments will reduce the frequency of GAD and will help to prevent comorbid Major Depression.[3]

GAD is characterized by excessive, recurrent, and prolonged worry and anxiety over simple daily concerns and minor issues. Typically, the focus of the anxiety shifts from one issue to another—unlike phobias, where the source(s) of anxiety remains consistent. Patients are usually aware that their concerns are disproportionate and sometimes ridiculous, but they are not able to change how they feel or think. The daily anxiety is so prominent that it interferes with concentration, attention, short-term memory, decision making, and confidence—people do not trust themselves to do what they need to do. It becomes impossible to conduct normal activities such as work, school, socializing with family and friends, and maintaining significant relationships. Those who live with GAD continuously over a long period of time begin to feel normal in that state, but they feel that there is nothing they can do to change it. Unfortunately, people with GAD often turn to alcohol or drugs to mask or manage their anxiety, and it is often the substance abuse that brings them into professional treatment.[4]

A diagnosis of GAD requires the following criteria:

1. Excessive anxiety and worry occurring most days over a continuous six-month period and involving a number of events or activities
2. The person's inability to control the worry
3. Anxiety and worry associated with at least three of the following (only one for children):
   a. Restlessness or feeling keyed up or on edge
   b. Easily fatigued
   c. Difficulty concentrating or feeling one's mind is blank
   d. Irritability
   e. Muscle tension
   f. Sleep disturbances
4. Anxiety or worry not confined to another Axis I disorder
5. Symptoms that cause significant distress or impairment in social, work, or other important areas of functioning
6. Disturbance is not due to direct impact of a substance or a medical condition and does not occur exclusively during a Mood Disorder, Psychotic Disorder, or other psychological disorder.[5]

Since everyone feels anxious at one time or another, there are specific criteria to differentiate between normal anxiety and GAD, but the main difference is the extreme distress and clear impairment in normal functioning found with GAD. More recent approaches to understanding GAD have led to a major revision in the way we view GAD, and that is to focus on worry as the primary defining quality. In addition to worrying about many different things, people with GAD can worry about worrying or even worry about not worrying! Some people will worry almost superstitiously, as if worrying will prevent the feared outcomes from happening.[6] GAD patients worry about family, personal finances, work, illness, and even minor things such as small mistakes or a social faux pas, and most will report that they typically worry at least half of every single day.[7] Children and teens are more likely to worry about school performance or performance in other areas like sports, music, or drama,[8] and children and teens can worry obsessively about potentially catastrophic events such as earthquakes, tornadoes, and asteroid strikes. They can also worry incessantly about contracting diseases such as AIDS, even though they have no risk factors, no exposure to anyone with AIDS, and have received considerable reassurance from family and physicians that they do not have the disease. These youngsters seem to need excessive reassurance about many things in their life, including their own physical or mental imperfections and inadequacies. They are often perfectionists and frequently complain about multiple physical problems. Children and teens with GAD usually act quite mature; are serious and reserved; and are often the eldest in small, competitive, achievement-oriented families.[9]

Most people with GAD complain about cognitive difficulties such as attention, concentration, and short-term memory as well as troubling thoughts and worries, and they typically manifest physical symptoms of anxiety such as muscle tension (especially in the neck and shoulders), headache (especially in the frontal and occipital areas), sweaty palms, shakiness, dryness of the mouth, palpitations, and difficulty breathing.[10] Many will report severe gastrointestinal symptoms, with about 30 percent having severe Irritable Bowel Syndrome.[11] Although chest pains are common in patients with Panic Disorder, they also exist in about 34 percent of patients with GAD who do not suffer from panic attacks.[12] Due to the myriad physical symptoms, patients with GAD tend to undergo many physical and laboratory tests to rule out physical disorders and ailments and have high medical service utilization rates.

Frequently, GAD is found to coexist with other disorders. Some comorbidities include:

1. Strong association with Major Depressive Disorder and Dysthymia
2. Low association with Panic Disorder—someone could have both GAD and PD, but it is not common
3. Hypomania, one of the characteristics of Bipolar II Disorder
4. Higher risk for suicide attempts
5. Treated more frequently and endure more frequent work impairments
6. Alcoholism, although not as common as in other Anxiety Disorders, and the pattern of abuse is often brief and nonpersistent.[10] It should be noted that when an alcohol-use disorder is present, GAD onset is typically later than the onset of the alcohol-use disorder.[13]

In summary, GAD is now considered a disorder of excessive and uncontrollable worry, a considerable shift from the earlier conceptualization found in the older *DSM-III-R*, which focused more on the somatic (physical) components of GAD symptoms. Worry and difficulties with cognitive processes now account for most of the symptoms that are identified as responsible for the pathogenesis (cause) and maintenance of this common and debilitating disorder.[14] Due to the new criteria, great strides in the last 20 years have improved both the diagnosis and treatment of GAD.[15] The new treatment forms include better medications, very effective psychotherapies, and even more use of common approaches such as exercise and relaxation techniques.[16]

Although most research reports a typical recovery rate of about 40 percent,[17] GAD remains one of the most difficult Anxiety Disorders to treat, even though it is a common, disabling, often chronic, and expensive condition.[18] Due to the variety of symptoms, multimodal treatment is often required, especially for the physical symptoms. Anxiolytic (antianxiety) medications and physical treatments such as deep muscle relaxation, meditation, and massage are often helpful, although not usually curative. The most common and successful treatments today involve cognitive-behavioral therapy, which often includes the use of relaxation techniques to reduce the amount and frequency of worrying. The precise relationship between muscle tension and GAD is not clear, but it is so common among GAD patients that it is often helpful to treat the tension with relaxation and other treatments such as massage.[17]

New treatments are emerging in the cognitive realm that address cognitive and behavioral symptoms. Patients with GAD preferentially attend to threat-relevant stimuli over neutral stimuli when both are present, and clinically anxious people with GAD consistently show an attentional bias toward threat. One study showed that GAD patients treated in an attention modification program showed a decrease in attentional bias to threat and a decrease in anxiety symptoms over the course of treatment.[18] This suggests that the treatment of GAD cannot simply attend to the physical symptoms but must focus on the cognitive and behavioral symptoms and that adequate treatment must deal with all of the symptom clusters, especially those most directly related to worry.

Panic Disorder

One of the most challenging and well-known Anxiety Disorders is Panic Disorder (PD). People who suffer from panic attacks experience severe and frightening symptoms such as pounding heart, trouble breathing, dizziness, chest pains, and nausea and usually report being in poorer physical health than the general population.[19] One of the characteristics of PD is being frightened by one's own physical symptoms, including the feeling that one is going to die or is going crazy. Panic attacks are the product of catastrophically misinterpreting autonomic arousal sensations that occur in the context of nonpathological anxiety as well as overreacting to other sources of arousal such as physical illness, exercise, and the ingestion of certain substances.[20] Experiencing an acute anxiety attack during or in association with a real physical threat is considered a fear reaction, and it is not the same as having a panic attack; a true panic attack occurs in the absence of any real danger.[21] Patients are rarely able to reliably predict when a panic attack will occur, although there are occasions when an attack may be expected and does occur. A panic attack can strike at any time, even during sleep, and usually lasts about 15 to 30 minutes. The symptoms will peak at about 10 minutes, although some of the residual symptoms may last longer. This unpredictability of an attack is quite significant to patients, since the fear of having another attack can be disabling in and of itself.

Anyone can experience a panic attack under the right circumstances, but to be diagnosed with Panic Disorder one must have experienced more than the occasional panic attack and must meet specific diagnostic criteria, although most people who experience a panic attack will never go on to develop Panic Disorder. One study found that the one-year prevalence rate for any type of panic attack (either unexpected or situationally caused) was about 28 percent, which means that more than one-quarter of the population will experience an attack during a given year, but the majority will never develop Panic Disorder.[22]

Panic Disorder occurs in six million Americans annually, affecting about twice as many women as men, although the clinical features, such as number and severity of symptoms, are much the same across the sexes.[23] PD typically appears in late adolescence or young adulthood, and a genetic connection gives relatives of patients with PD the probability of developing it. It does not mean, however, that if a family member has been diagnosed with Panic Disorder, you will develop it as well. More current models of Panic Disorder focus on the fear-of-anxiety construct, suggesting that there is a learning component to the disorder.[24] In the expectancy model of fear, panic attacks result from having the predisposition to catastrophically misinterpret and to respond with fear to benign sensations of arousal and from possessing a learned fear of anxiety, which is continually maintained by experiencing panic episodes.[25] Some believe that this vicious cycle first begins with anything that can cause arousal and then leads to a misinterpretation of emerging physical symptoms; second, anxiety emerges and accelerates to the point of panic; and, finally, the person learns to fear the original cause of arousal as well as any other situations where a similar arousal might occur.[24]

Panic Disorder is diagnosed in about 10 percent of patients seen at mental health clinics and in 10 percent to 60 percent of patients seen in various medical specialty clinics (e.g., cardiology and pulmonology).[26] The National Comorbidity Study found a lifetime prevalence rate of Panic Disorder in the general population of 3.5 percent,[27] although most other studies found life-time prevalence rates in the range of 1 percent to 2 percent. Generally, the prevalence rates are fairly consistent around the world.[28] The age of onset of PD is distributed bimodally, with typical onset occurring between 15 to 19 years and 25 to 30 years of age.[29] As mentioned earlier, many people with PD suffer from Agoraphobia, or the fear of being in unfamiliar or unsafe situations. From the sparse data collected, it appears that Agoraphobia affects about 0.6 percent of older adults (ages 55 to 65) in any 12-month period, al-though most patients report that it begins earlier. PD is rarely found in people over age 65, and, as in younger samples, it affects twice as many women as men. Married people are less likely to develop Agoraphobia, but the loss of a spouse and the onset of other health and/or psychological problems may precipitate PD.[30]

The frequency of attacks varies considerably in individuals with Panic Disorder, and those who experience repeated panic attacks can become disabled by restricting activities and avoiding situations for fear of having a panic attack and then developing Agoraphobia. In clinical samples, PD with Agoraphobia is more common than PD without it. If Panic Disorder is diagnosed early, before Agoraphobia develops, it is one of the most treatable Anxiety Disorders; however, some patients go from one doctor to another trying to find help and answers (often called "doctor shopping") and may rely on other delaying factors such as cancelling appointments and going to nonmedical and nonpsychological providers for assistance. Unfortunately, these delays tend to prevent timely and appropriate treatment. Treatment usually involves medications in conjunction with psychotherapy in order to address the cognitive and behavioral symptoms of PD. One complicating factor is that PD is frequently comorbid with conditions such as Depression, drug abuse, or alcoholism.[31] PD with or without Agoraphobia is also associated with a poor overall quality of life as well as impaired occupational, scholastic, and social functioning. As a highly treatable condition, it is important to recognize, diagnose, and treat PD early and adequately. Without treatment, PD and Agoraphobia may wax and wane, but they both appear to be chronic conditions.[32]

A diagnosis of PD will specify whether it is with or without Agoraphobia; otherwise, the criteria are exactly the same. Someone with PD will have at least four of the following symptoms:

1. Rapid heart beat
2. Sweating
3. Shortness of breath
4. Choking feeling or feeling of being smothered
5. Dizziness
6. Nausea
7. Feelings of unreality

8. Numbness
9. Hot flashes or chills
10. Chest pain
11. Fear of dying
12. Fear of going insane

The diagnostic criteria for PD with Agoraphobia are:

1. Both (a) and (b):
   a. Recurrent and unexpected panic attacks
   b. At least one of the attacks has been followed by one month or more of:
      I. Persistent concern about having another attack
      II. Worry about the implications of the attack or its consequences (e.g., losing control, having a heart attack, going crazy)
2. Presence of agoraphobia
3. Panic attacks are not a result of the direct physical effects of a substance (e.g., a drug of abuse or medication) or a general medical condition
4. Panic attacks are not better accounted for by another mental disorder, including other Anxiety Disorders.[5]

The diagnostic criteria for Agoraphobia are:

1. Anxiety about being in places or situations from which escape might be difficult or embarrassing, or where help may not be available during a panic attack; usually fears different clusters of situations and venturing into them, with the number increasing over time.
2. Situations are avoided or endured with marked distress and worry about having a panic attack or similar symptoms. Confronting difficult situations is usually aided by the presence of a companion.
3. Anxiety or avoidance is not better accounted for by another mental disorder.[5]

One requirement for PD is that unexpected panic attacks occur without any obvious causal factor; however, not all attacks are unexpected.[24] Interestingly, some patients do not experience a fearful response as a result of a panic attack. About 30 percent of panic attacks occur without the fear of dying or going crazy, and these patients do not differ in terms of age, age of onset, or frequency from those who experience attacks with feelings of fear. Due to the lack of fear, the attacks are rarely associated with shortness of breath, trembling, smothering, and depersonalization, and patients are less likely to experience anticipatory anxiety or be treated with medication, although frequency of attacks leads to the same rate of diagnosis and functional disability. Further, these patients are less likely to develop Agoraphobia or other Axis I disorders such as Major Depression. Depending upon how a patient reports his symptoms, the absence of a fear response during panic attacks may lead to the mistaken assumption that the PD is less severe.[33]

Risk factors for PD include gender, since women are twice as susceptible to develop PD, and marital status, a significant risk factor since the highest lifetime prevalence rates are reported for widowed, separated, or divorced people. No consistent findings relate PD to educational level, and some have found a relationship between smoking and PD, but the causal link is unclear. Sometimes an understandable link between Pulmonary Disease and PD is reported, since breathing problems can trigger panic attacks.

The most common of comorbid Anxiety Disorders (not including Agoraphobia, since it is an element of the diagnosis) are: Social Phobia, GAD, Obsessive-Compulsive Disorder, and Posttraumatic Stress Disorder. Between 30 percent and 60 percent of patients with PD will also suffer from a Depressive Disorder, and about 36 percent will suffer from Substance Abuse, often using alcohol or drugs to self-medicate, although recent evidence suggests that abuse usually begins prior to the development of Panic Disorder. Some epidemiology studies demonstrate that Major Depressive Disorder occurs in up to 56 percent of patients with PD at some point in their life, and in approximately two-thirds of these cases, the symptoms of Depression develop along with or secondary to PD. However, since Major Depression usually precedes the PD, it cannot be assumed that the Depression is always a reaction to the PD. Medical conditions that are likely to be comorbid with PD include cardiac, gastrointestinal, respiratory, and neurological diseases.[34]

Experiencing a panic attack is terrifying and is a primary reason that people seek emergency department consultations.[35] Frequent emergency room visits are one of the reasons why PD sufferers generate high medical expenses; these patients also tend to undergo costly medical tests to rule out other medical problems.[36] PD is also a leading cause for people seeking mental health services, surpassing both Schizophrenia and Mood Disorders.[37] Typically, people do not begin their search for help by contacting mental health professionals but are referred by a physician who has no medical explanation for the patient's symptoms.[38]

Seasonal and meteorological changes affect people with PD similarly to those with Seasonal Affective Disorder (SAD). The frequency of panic attacks varies by month, usually increasing in August and December; although, if a patient peaks in August, she typically will not increase in December and vice versa. Panic attacks are also more likely to occur during cloudy weather, during hot or cold extremes, and when it is humid.[39]

Although PD is a highly treatable condition, especially if caught early, it is not usually recognized and diagnosed accurately in the primary care setting, which can lead to unnecessary and costly diagnostic procedures as well as inappropriate referrals to cardiologists. In one study, medical specialists were given a survey to determine their knowledge of panic attacks and the availability of effective treatments. The results are as follows:

- 51 percent answered the knowledge-based questions correctly.
- Most knew the definition of a panic attack but knew little about its clinical features or treatment.
- 97.4 percent believed medication effectively relieves panic symptoms.
- 32.5 percent knew that cognitive-behavioral therapy is a first-line treatment for Panic Disorder.
- 6 percent knew how to implement cognitive-behavioral therapy with their patients.
- 56.1 percent recognized that psychologists could effectively treat Panic Disorder.[40]

Although the typical treatment for PD includes medication, medication is rarely adequate alone and must be coupled with other types of psychological treatment. Cognitive-behavioral therapy is the approach that receives the most support because it offers a variety of behavioral and cognitive strategies to minimize the symptoms of panic.

New types of treatment are being introduced and evaluated, including panic-focused psychodynamic psychotherapy (PFPP), which is based on older forms of treatment dating back to Freud's psychoanalysis. Since the traditional psychodynamic approaches often take longer and are difficult to evaluate, they are rarely used. However, newer and briefer forms of psychodynamic treatments such as PFPP are being used and are proving effective in treating PD. With such developments, the psychoanalytic type of therapy can be systematically evaluated in a mode consistent with the principles of evidence-based medicine.[41]

Identifying what triggers panic attacks is of primary importance to those who experience them. Unfortunately, the proximal cause of a panic attack is rarely found in the immediate situation but rather in the accumulation of many experiences over time. Regardless of whether a person is diagnosed with PD, it is important to remember that the panic attack itself does not pose any real physical danger. When someone experiences a panic attack, he needs to mentally accept the fact that it is happening and not try to fight the symptoms; the attack will usually subside within 10 to 20 minutes. As simple as this sounds, it is, in fact, very difficult for someone who is in the middle of a panic attack to think rationally. If the person can ride it out rather than become more upset, the panic attack will subside more quickly. It is also important to recognize the early warning signs of a panic attack, because practicing some effective techniques (e.g., regulated breathing) can stop or minimize the attack. Sometimes people can abruptly tell themselves to "Stop It" and immediately focus on something other than themselves as a means of shortening or lessening the impact of an attack—this works best if it is done early. Finally, if someone experiences four or more attacks during a month and/or the fear of having another attack becomes disruptive to one's life, it is time to seek professional help from a specialist who is experienced in treating PD.

SUMMARY

Generalized Anxiety Disorder and Panic Disorder involve different symptom patterns and are treated with different techniques and modalities. GAD is characterized by lower levels of and more diffuse types of anxiety and worry that emerge in varying degrees most of the time and on most days. PD involves acute and intense periods of anxiety that do not last long but are frightening and can be incapacitating. The fear of future panic attacks can severely limit activities and the quality of life for patients. These two Anxiety Disorders share similarities as well, and are both are characterized by anxiety, although the type of anxiety experienced is generally quite different. Most importantly, both conditions respond well to medications and psychotherapies, especially when diagnosed and treated early, making it critical that providers at the primary care level (where these disorders are typically first seen) understand and recognize the symptoms of GAD and PD and make appropriate, timely referrals.

6

Types of Anxiety Disorders II: Phobias, Posttraumatic Stress Disorder, and Obsessive-Compulsive Disorder

> How can you diagnose . . . obsessive-compulsive disorder, and then act like I have some choice about barging in here?
> —Jack Nicholson as the character Melvin Udall talking to his psychiatrist in the movie *As Good As It Gets*

In addition to Generalized Anxiety Disorder (GAD) and Panic Disorder (PD), there are several other anxiety-based conditions that include Specific and Social Phobias, Posttraumatic Stress Disorder (PTSD), Acute Stress Disorder, and Obsessive-Compulsive Disorder (OCD). These disorders differ from GAD and PD but unquestionably involve and are identified with anxiety as well.

PHOBIAS

Phobia is the most identifiable and understandable of the Anxiety Disorders when it involves common fears such as snakes or dangerous animals, but other feared objects or situations, though not as obvious, are also identified. The following list includes the names of some unusual (but real) Phobias:

Ablutophobia—Fear of washing or bathing
Alektorophobia—Fear of chickens
Anemophobia—Fear of air drafts or wind
Arachibutyrophobia—Fear of peanut butter sticking to the roof of the mouth
Barophobia—Fear of gravity
Bogyphobia—Fear of bogies or the bogeyman
Bromidrosiphobia—Fear of body smells

Chronophobia—Fear of time
Decidophobia—Fear of making decisions
Dutchphobia—Fear of the Dutch
Hedonophobia—Fear of feeling pleasure
Hippopotomonstrosesquippedaliophobia—Fear of long words
Lachanophobia—Fear of vegetables
Melissaphobia—Fear of bees
Opthalmophobia—Fear of being stared at
Parthenophobia—Fear of virgins
Sophophobia—Fear of learning
Teratophobia—Fear of giving birth to a monster; or fear of deformed people or
   monsters
Walloonphobia—Fear of Walloons (a group of French-speaking people living in
   the south of Belgium)
Xylophobia—Fear of wooden objects or forests

Many of the fears listed here seem harmless and are good examples of how anxiety is formed using the two-factor learning theory. A fear is learned when a neutral object becomes the source of a Phobia through classical conditioning, followed by avoidance learning, which produces a reward of decreased anxiety (negative reinforcement) as the person avoids or escapes the feared object. In addition to the learning component, new research has demonstrated that disgust plays a role in the development of animal fears and phobias, and this is particularly true in the acquisition and avoidance elements.[1]

Mild fears of certain objects are not unusual or pathological, but irrational or disproportionate fears warrant a diagnosis of Phobia—particularly when the fear causes significant distress or impairs the person socially, occupationally, or educationally. Children will pass through different developmental stages, which often include being fearful of various things, but most will gradually outgrow their fears without a problem. My twin daughters experienced a phase at about age three when they were afraid of helicopters. If they heard a helicopter overhead while playing outside, they would run into the garage until the sound of the helicopter went away. If they were playing inside, they would look up in search of the sound but did not seem concerned. Thus, the fear of helicopters was specific to being outdoors when not safely under cover. I have no idea where this fear originated, but it disappeared within a few weeks.

Some childhood fears continue into adulthood and occasionally become diagnostically relevant. For example, my sister is afraid of bugs and insists that her fear is due to early learning and the actions of her brother (me), who frequently scared her with bugs when we were children. Since neither of our parents feared bugs, I suppose her theory is valid. This Phobia of bugs is clearly a learned fear reaction, but it does not disrupt my sister's life enough to warrant treatment. To qualify for the diagnosis of Phobia, there must be a *per-*

sistent, irrational fear and *avoidance* of the specific thing or activity that elicits the fear. Further, the diagnosis is only offered when the Phobia impairs the individual's social, occupational, educational, or other important functioning.

Generally, Phobias are listed in three groups: Agoraphobia, Specific Phobia, and Social Phobia. Agoraphobia, the fear of going out to other places, was discussed in chapter 5 along with Panic Disorder. Specific Phobias are common and rarely require treatment because they seldom significantly disrupt a person's life. Common types of Specific Phobias involve animals such as spiders, snakes, mice, rats, and dogs. Other types include fears of flying, heights, injections, public transportation, confined spaces, dentists, storms, tunnels, and bridges. Although some of these fears can be disruptive, it is a testimony to a person's creativity as to how they avoid the objects they fear and still manage to function normally. Famous sports announcer John Madden is afraid to fly, so he travels around the country in a huge, luxurious motor home. A patient of mine who is retired and spends most of the winter in the South is also afraid to fly. He uses the Auto Train to transport himself and his car south and drives when returning north. I offered to treat his fear of flying (pterygophobia), but he declined, saying that he liked and would continue the arrangements even if he was not afraid to fly.

The last major type of Phobia is Social Phobia, which includes Generalized Social Phobia and Specific (or Discrete) Social Phobia. In both cases, the person becomes severely anxious while in general or specific types of social situations.

Specific Phobias

Phobias are among the most common mental disorders;[2] among a large community sample in the Epidemiological Catchment Area study, there was a lifetime prevalence of 11.25 percent for Specific Phobias and 2.73 percent for Social Phobia.[3] The National Comorbidity Study found a lifetime prevalence rate for Specific Phobias of 11.30 percent in a sample of 8,000 people across the United States. It is estimated that about 19.2 million American adults suffer from some type of Phobia, with twice as many women as men being diagnosed with Specific Phobia. This is particularly true of animal phobias, although there are fewer differences between the sexes for acrophobia (fear of heights) and trypanophobia (fear of blood injections). Typically, Phobias emerge in childhood or adolescence and persist into adulthood, but they are not the same as normal, developmental childhood fears. Also, Phobias tend to run in families and are assumed to be the result of observational or other forms of learning.[4]

Specific Phobias are circumscribed (very specific), persistent, and unreasonable fears of a particular object or situation and are the second most common

Anxiety Disorder after Social Phobia. Although Specific Phobias tend to be less incapacitating than other Anxiety Disorders, the person usually recognizes the fear as unrealistic, and most people with Specific Phobias are able adjust their lifestyle to completely avoid or minimize contact with the feared object.[5] Some intense Phobias are so circumscribed that the person can perform certain tasks in specific situations that seem potentially fearful. For example, trained pilots with severe acrophobia may be unable to climb a step-ladder, or athletes who ski the highest mountains may not be able to look off the side of a bridge. This may seem irrational, but the very nature of a Phobia is that the fear is irrational. Recall from chapter 1 that the fear of a loss of control is often included with feelings of anxiety. Pilots have control of their planes and skiers are in control of themselves as they head down a slope; therefore, they do not notice the heights while they are performing because they feel in control of the situation.

A person with a genuine Phobia who is forced to face the feared object or situation will usually experience acute anxiety and even a panic attack. However, if the patient seldom encounters the feared object (e.g., snakes), he may not bother to pursue treatment since the Phobia does not adversely affect his daily life. It is encouraging to note that treatment for Phobias is usually successful, and Specific Phobias respond very well to psychotherapies that focus on the fears and ways to reduce them.[2]

Research during the last decade has resulted in more effective treatments for both Social and Specific Phobias. Specific Phobias tend to co-occur with other Specific Phobias, and in one sample 76 percent of patients with a lifetime history of Specific Phobias reported one or more co-occurring Phobias.[6] For example, 70 percent of people with hemophobia (fear of blood) have injection Phobias as well.[7] However, there are exceptions, and while the clustering of Phobias is interesting, it is not likely to be helpful from a theoretical or treatment standpoint.[2]

Social Phobia

Social Phobia is a common problem that is frequently underdiagnosed and undertreated. It may emerge as a generalized type of Phobia, where people are fearful in most social situations, or as a nongeneralized type (usually called Discrete or Specific Social Phobia), which focuses on only one or two situations that are usually related to public performance of some kind.[8] Social Phobia affects about 15 million American adults (6.8% of the population). It produces undue embarrassment and anxiety in social situations and is extreme enough to impair normal social functioning.[9] In this particular type of Phobia, women tend to predominate but not by much.[10] Men are more fearful than women of urinating in public bathrooms and of returning items to a store, whereas women are more fearful of talking to people in authority, public speaking, being the center of attention, expressing disagreement, and throwing a party.[11]

People with Social Phobia are extremely self-conscious when in social situations, fear being watched and judged by others, and fear doing something embarrassing. They may worry and obsess for days or weeks prior to doing something, regardless of being aware that their fears are unrealistic and unreasonable. Even if they succeed at doing something that they fear, they will worry excessively before the event, be nervous during it, and then worry for hours afterward about what they did, how they did, and how people may have judged them.[4]

Social Phobia can be limited to one or a few situations or generalized to any social situation, but it is a condition that displays many of the physical symptoms of anxiety. It usually emerges in childhood or adolescence and persists into adulthood. Some have proposed that a genetic factor is involved, but this is still unclear, and the mechanisms of action are not well understood.[4] Social Phobia tends to run in families; the rate is three times higher in patients' families than in the general population. While observational learning and other learning processes may be responsible, a higher concordance of Social Phobia in monozygotic (identical) than dizygotic (fraternal) twins implies a genetic process.[12]

Questions about the relationship between shyness and Social Phobia persist, but they are not the same issues at all. One study looked at shy people with and without Social Phobia as well as non-shy people with and without Social Phobia. In both the shy and non-shy groups, people with Social Phobia reported more symptomatology, more functional impairment, and a lower quality of life than those without Social Phobia. About one-third of highly shy people without Social Phobia reported no social fears at all. Shy people without Social Phobia and socially phobic subjects both reported similar levels of anxiety in normal conversation, but the socially phobic group reported more anxiety during the task of giving a speech, and the Social Phobia subjects performed less effectively than those without Social Phobia across all tasks.[13] Clearly, Social Phobia is not just a severe case of shyness.

The anxiety associated with Social Phobia can be so intense that it may lead to physical reactions such as blushing, stammering, sweating, gastrointestinal upset, racing heart, trembling limbs, and even a full-scale panic attack. These physical symptoms can evoke intense emotions that are hidden most of the time, and the physical reactions that are experienced often produce additional embarrassment and humiliation. One of the main challenges is the intrusive nature of the symptoms, which can interfere with important areas of a person's functioning. For example, in one music school, 16 percent of the students said that performance anxiety had limited their careers, and at an international conference of symphony and opera musicians, 24 percent said that they had suffered seriously from stage fright.[12]

Social Phobia is a common diagnosis that may affect 1 percent to 13 percent of the population, depending on how the Phobia is defined. If we look at the most serious variants of this disorder, it is more likely that about 1 percent to 2 percent of the population experiences significant impairment of work and/or social life. During one phone survey, 21 percent of the respondents said that they try to avoid public speaking, and 17 percent said that they try to avoid eating in a restaurant. Another 3 percent try to avoid writing in public, and 0.2 percent said they consistently avoid urinating in public restrooms. In this sample, 2 percent experienced significant distress during more than one of these situations.[12]

In terms of comorbidities, Social Phobia frequently co-occurs with other disorders: 59 percent of patients with Social Phobia also had another Specific Phobia, 49 percent had Panic Disorder with Agoraphobia, 19 percent were alcohol abusers (often self-medicating to reduce the anxiety), 17 percent suffered from Major Depressive Disorder, and 10–20percent of people in clinics for treatment of Anxiety Disorders also had Social Phobia, the most common diagnosis for a person with another Anxiety Disorder. Major Depression is often associated with Social Phobia, and family members of patients with Social Phobia experience a high rate of Depression. One study showed that patients with Social Phobia and Panic Disorder had a 95percent risk of also developing Major Depression, and another study showed that alcoholics have nine times the average rate of Social Phobia.[12] Generalized Social Phobia is associated with Depression, Anxiety, general distress, and concerns about negative evaluation from others, and Discrete Social Phobia seems to be associated with greater cardiac reactivity,[14] which means that people with Discrete Social Phobia show more changes in heart rhythms when under stress and this is an indication of how their bodies react to stressful situations. It is important to determine whether a person with a cardiac condition also suffers from Discrete Social Phobia, because treatment would be necessary for both conditions.

Generalized Social Phobia is pervasive and persistent and closely resembles Avoidant Personality Disorder (APD), but the qualities of the two disorders are quite different. Patients with APD are hypersensitive to criticism and rejection and do not express their feelings for fear of ridicule. They want affection and closeness with others but will do nothing to get it. They are afraid to start conversations, ask questions, make friends, or join groups. They consider themselves inept or inferior, and they are often depressed. One major difference between APD and Social Phobia is that patients with APD do not have the anxiety component; or, if they have anxiety, it is minimally intrusive and not clinically significant.[12]

In terms of a differential diagnosis, Social Phobia must be distinguished from other disorders as well as APD, because there are additional disorders that involve fear and avoidance of specific situations. For example, Panic Disorder with Agoraphobia can certainly look like Social Phobia or even a situationally based Specific Phobia. PTSD also presents similarly to Social or Specific Phobia, but the key is that the symptoms of PTSD follow the traumatic event and would not have been present prior to it. Obsessive-Compulsive Disorder may resemble Social or Specific Phobia until one reviews a complete clinical picture of all the symptoms. Finally, as mentioned above, any type of Phobia must be separated from normal fears and shyness.[2] To make a proper differential diagnosis, a careful history and a thorough evaluation are essential.

POSTTRAUMATIC STRESS DISORDER AND ACUTE STRESS DISORDER

"It could go on for years and years, and has, for centuries," wrote the author of the Sumerian *Epic of Gilgamesh* in the third millennium BC, describing the suffering of one of the characters who survived a violent episode that killed his friend.[15] History contains numerous examples of the damaging and lasting effects of severe trauma. Although the diagnosis of Posttraumatic Stress Disorder is fairly recent, the phenomenon to which it refers is well known and has been documented for centuries with various names. We are, however, just beginning to fully understand and appreciate the complexity of this disorder, although some still question its validity. It is not surprising that most references to the realities of warfare include descriptions of the horrific events that people have experienced, but some believe that PTSD is not a true condition but rather an invention meant only highlight the political point that war is harmful to mental health. I suggest that skeptics would benefit from volunteering their time at a veterans hospital and helping with military men and women who have experienced the horrors of combat and are now suffering from PTSD. Posttraumatic Stress Disorder is a very real disorder with very real casualties, and people who dismiss it or minimize it are poorly informed, have their own political agenda, or both.

In the aftermath of wars in recent decades, mental health professionals have come to recognize that some military personnel have experienced events so traumatic that the person is severely and sometimes permanently affected. During the Civil War, this condition was known as "battle fatigue," which implied a temporary condition based upon the cumulative effects of being in combat. In World War I, it was called "shell shock," a term that evolved due to the increased use of artillery and to soldiers hiding in trenches, hoping that shells would not fall and kill them. Doctors during World War II began to recognize the psychopathological nature of soldiers' reactions to being in combat by labeling it "combat neurosis" or "traumatic neurosis." Even with an increased level of understanding, it was still assumed that people who suffered from this condition were emotionally and psychologically weak or inadequate. Hence, the famous scene in the movie *Patton* when Gen. George Patton slaps a soldier, who was removed from the front for combat neurosis, and calls him a coward. Although Patton was reprimanded for his actions and publically apologized, his actions represented the typical reaction of most people when they saw or heard about a trauma-related condition—this did not happen to "strong" people.[15]

During the Korean War, the *DSM-I* was created (in 1952) to coordinate and standardize efforts to diagnose mental illnesses, and this trauma-induced condition was initially called a "gross stress reaction." This was the first war in U.S. history when psychological factors were given serious attention. Brain-washing and other forms of psychological warfare during this conflict, as well as movies like *The Manchurian Candidate*, increased interest in the topic. When the *DSM-II* was published (1969), this condition was labeled "transient situational disturbance," finally acknowledging the probability that the stress and trauma of a situation was at the root of a psychological condition. The Vietnam conflict led to an increased awareness of PTSD and introduced to the public the use of the term PTSD for this disorder.[15]

As part of my early training, I worked in a veterans hospital during the Vietnam War and saw the casualties. Most of the military personnel never spoke about their experiences and swore they never would. This was also true of my father's friends who survived World War II; as a youngster I was interested in hearing their stories, but few of them had anything to say about their experiences and the men clearly wanted to leave their memories in the remote past.

Although the earliest focus on PTSD was concerned with the military, much of recent research has been conducted on victims of crime, including sexual assault and rape, as well as victims of natural disasters and catastrophic events such as the September 11, 2001, terrorist attacks. In general, three types of symptoms are seen with PTSD:

1. Hyperarousal
   a. Irritability
   b. Increased startle reaction
   c. Hypervigilance
   d. Sleep difficulties
   e. Concentration problems
2. Re-experiencing or intrusion
   a. Vivid memories
   b. Nightmares

    c. Re-experiencing the event

    d. Anything that reminds the person of the trauma is troubling

3. Avoidance and emotional numbing

    a. Avoidance of feelings, thoughts, persons, places, and situations that evoke the memories

    b. Loss of interest in usual activities

    c. Feeling estranged from others and even from one's own feelings

    d. Common themes—fixation on the trauma

PTSD is now routinely recognized in places where natural disasters, war, and catastrophic events occur. Community-based studies find a lifetime prevalence rate of 8 percent in the adult population,[16] and women are twice as likely to experience PTSD.[17] The highest rates of PTSD (one-third to three-fourths of those exposed to trauma) are found among rape survivors, military combat personnel, prisoners of war, those performing graves registration duties (people responsible for retrieving dead bodies after a battle), and those who have experienced ethnically and politically motivated internment and genocide.[17] PTSD is often a chronic condition with a significant number of people remaining symptomatic several years following the initial traumatic event and rarely making a full recovery.[2] In fact, at least one-third of those diagnosed with PTSD fail to recover even after many years.[16]

The diagnostic criteria for PTSD include:

1. The person has been exposed to a traumatic event that includes both (a) and (b):

    a. The person experienced, witnessed, or was confronted with an event or events that involved actual or threatened death or serious injury, or a threat to the self or others.

    b. The person's response involved intense fear, feelings of helplessness, or horror (in children this may be expressed as disorganized or agitated behavior).

2. The traumatic event is re-experienced in one or more of the following ways:

    a. Recurrent distressing thoughts or perceptions (children may act out some of the trauma in play activities)

    b. Nightmares about the trauma (children may have more vague nightmares)

    c. Reliving the event through flashbacks, ruminations, and obsessions (children may reenact the trauma)

    d. Intense psychological distress when confronted by anything that reminds the person of the trauma

    e. Physiological reactivity to stimuli related to the trauma

3. Persistent avoidance and numbing of general responsiveness (three or more of the following):

    a. Avoidance of thoughts, feelings, or conversations about the trauma

    b. Avoidance of people, activities, and places that remind the person of the trauma

    c. Inability to recall things about the trauma

    d. Diminished interest in participating in significant activities

    e. Feelings of detachment or estrangement from others

    f. Restricted range of affect

    g. Sense of a foreshortened future

4. Persistent symptoms of increased arousal that were not there before the trauma. At least two of the following symptoms must persist for at least one month and must cause significant distress and/or problems in important areas of functioning:

    a. Difficulty falling asleep or staying asleep

    b. Irritability and/or angry outbursts

    c. Problems with concentration

    d. Hypervigilence

    e. Increased startle response

5. Must also specify if:

    a. Acute—duration less than three months

    b. Chronic—duration more than three months

    c. Delayed onset—at least six months after the trauma[18]

One difficulty in diagnosing PTSD is that some people can experience symptoms similar to PTSD without experiencing a traumatic event—at least as defined in the diagnostic criteria. One study showed that trauma rarely led to PTSD in children and adolescents, but the rates of other psychiatric disorders nearly doubled following a traumatic event. Obviously, people can be significantly impacted by a trauma but may not develop PTSD.[15]

Many people experience symptoms of dissociation following a trauma (e.g., amnesia, feelings of detachment or estrangement, depersonalization or derealization), and discussions continue about whether dissociative phenomena should be included in the diagnostic criteria for PTSD. However, since these symptoms are not found universally in PTSD patients, it is questionable whether they should be considered. Controversy also persists about the existence of "partial PTSD," when a person has most but not all of the criteria to qualify for the diagnosis. It seems that these individuals are in need of treatment just as someone who has all of the necessary criteria.[19]

In recent years there have been discussions about what is considered traumatic. PTSD is defined as much by the etiology (the causes) as the phenomenology (the meaning to the person experiencing it). To qualify for the diagnosis of PTSD the person must experience an event that meets the criteria mentioned in the *DSM-IV* that are listed earlier. However, as specific as these criteria sound, there is still room for interpretation. Community-based studies have shown that 70 percent of people will experience at least one traumatic event during the course of their lives.[20] Many have assumed, and with some support, that there is a relationship between the magnitude of the event and the risk of developing PTSD.[21] While this makes sense, an individual's cognitive and affective responses to the trauma are also significant in determining the risk of PTSD.[21] Even some people who have received a serious medical diagnosis have demonstrated the necessary criteria for PTSD,[22] and witnessing medical events can be traumatic.[2]

Defining what is traumatic is fraught with challenges because of the variability in responses on the part of each person. Recently, we have seen a shift away from focusing on the traumatic event to more consideration for the response of the person—what is traumatic to one person may not be to another. Further, we continue to redefine what is meant by a traumatic event, and each consecutive edition of the *DSM* has broadened the concept of trauma. It is now apparent that many more people have been exposed to trauma than was originally thought.[19] I was asked to be an expert witness in a trial that involved a person claiming to have developed PTSD as a result of a workplace accident. While performing his job this person came in contact with a chemical that he thought was toxic and deadly; he was significantly traumatized and believed that he was going to die. No one could identify the chemical or the treatment required, and it was quite some time before it was determined that the chemical was not immediately dangerous and did not pose a threat to the health, well-being, and life of the employee. The defense claimed that the chemical was not deadly and, therefore, was not a significant traumatic event. My testimony stressed that the experienced trauma was based on the perception of the employee at the time of the event and that PTSD symptoms were present more than a month later. Discovering later that the chemical was not fatal was obviously a relief, but it was not a cure for the already existing disorder. The court agreed, and the claim for damages was recognized.

Determining the extent of trauma within a population depends upon the criteria used to define it. Using a broad definition of trauma, the National Institute of Mental Health Epidemiologic Catchment Area study found that 60 percent of men and 50 percent of women had experienced trauma.[15] Clearly, the vast majority of people who experience trauma do not go on to develop PTSD, and one large German study found that 90 percent of women and 97 percent of men who experience trauma do not develop PTSD. More than two-thirds of children had experienced a traumatic event, and one-third had experienced more than one—often by hearing of something that had happened to someone else. Of these children, only 13 percent had any symptoms of PTSD, and 1 in 200 had PTSD itself.[15]

Depending upon the study, women are two to three times more likely than men to develop PTSD due to the different types of trauma that women are exposed to. Men tend to experience trauma that is nonsexual physical violence, and women experience trauma that more often involves rape and childhood sexual abuse, which may occur over a longer period of time and can have a more profound, long-lasting effect. Of men and women who experience the same event, women are more likely to develop PTSD,[15] although it has not been easy to determine why this occurs. A recent study by Nydegger et al.[23] reports that, among career professional firefighters, the longer a person had been on the job, the greater the probability he had experienced PTSD or at least developed some PTSD symptoms. The study also determined that firefighters rarely sought professional help and tended to rely more on humor, emotional support, avoidance, and alcohol use to manage their symptoms. Therefore, several questions are left to answer: Are men less likely to develop PTSD or are they less likely to report it and seek help or, perhaps, both? It is possible that women are better at soothing and supporting men after a traumatic event than men are at comforting women.[15] The Nydegger et al. study implies that, without treatment, the effects of PTSD worsen over time for some people.[23] This is consistent with findings reported on Gulf War veterans that showed an increase in symptoms of PTSD over time, with 3 percent showing signs of PTSD immediately after the war and more than 8 percent showing significant symptoms two years later. However, it was also found that of people who experienced symptoms of PTSD following a trauma, 58 percent of them sought professional help and reported a 36-months-to-remission rate compared to a 64-months-to-remission rate for those who did not get help.[24]

In addition to exposure to trauma, other factors seem to be related to one's vulnerability for developing PTSD. For example, PTSD is more likely to affect someone who has experienced prior traumatic events and intentional injury (e.g., physical or sexual assault) than someone who has experienced natural disasters, and this is especially true if the victim feels at fault for the trauma. Some studies have shown that having a high IQ may blunt the effects of a traumatic event, but having a low IQ tends to increase the intensity of the response. Increased vulnerability to PTSD is also caused by depression, anxiety, alcohol and drug abuse, childhood behavior disorders, adolescent delinquency, Antisocial Personality Disorder, and other Personality Disorders. One German study found that firefighters who had less confidence in their own abilities and were more hostile were also more likely to develop PTSD.[15] Twin and adoption studies suggest a genetic factor in determining one's susceptibility to PTSD. Research evidence reveals that some people are concerned about patients faking PTSD symptoms in order to obtain disability benefits;[15] while this is a valid concern, it is not likely to include a large number of people. In another study, men and women who volunteered for a study on Depression revealed that 80 percent had experienced a traumatic event that fit the criteria for PTSD. It is likely that the *DSM-V* will redefine PTSD to focus less on the traumatic events and more on the reactions of people and their vulnerabilities before and after the trauma.[15]

There is evidence that what occurs following the traumatic event may be as important as what happens before—at least in terms of developing PTSD.

The range of responses, support, vulnerability factors, and individual person-alities and differences all must be considered. It is not surprising that PTSD is frequently misdiagnosed due to its complexity. Some of the reasons are:

- High rate of comorbidity
- Patient denial or misrepresentation
- Overly high diagnostic thresholds set by clinicians
- Failure to take a trauma history[24]

Complicating both the diagnosis and treatment of PTSD are the high rates of comorbidity. Studies reveal a lifetime comorbidity rate of PTSD with at least one psychiatric disorder is 88 percent in men and 79 percent in women. The most common comorbid conditions are:

- Mood Disorders (50% for Major Depression, 20% for Dysthymia)
- Other Anxiety Disorders (16% Generalized Anxiety Disorder, 9% Panic Disorder, 30% Specific Phobia, 28% Social Phobia, 19% Ago-raphobia)
- Substance Use Disorders (52% alcohol abuse in men, 34% drug abuse in men, 28% alcohol abuse in women, 27% drug abuse in women)
- Conduct Disorder (43% in men, 15% in women)[24]

The course of PTSD depends upon many factors. Immediately following a trauma, a high percentage of victims will develop a myriad of symptoms that can include disorganized behavior, dissociative symptoms, psychomo-tor changes, and occasional paranoid symptoms.[2] The range of outcomes in-cludes:

- Full recovery
- Relatively unchanging course with only mild fluctuations
- More obvious fluctuations with intermittent periods of well-being and recurrences of major symptoms
- Deterioration with age in a limited number of cases due to the passage of time with no resolution of symptoms
- Increased startle response, nightmares, irritability, and depression[2]

General medical conditions (e.g., head injury, burns, etc.) can also occur as a direct consequence of trauma. PTSD may be associated with the increased rate of adverse medical conditions such as musculoskeletal problems and car-diovascular morbidity,[25] further complicating the diagnosis, treatment, and prognosis. The course and outlook of PTSD are often uncertain; in one study, less than 28 percent of people who had witnessed a mass killing spree recovered within a year, and in another study of the same event, 46 percent of patients had developed chronic PTSD.[15] We are now aware that PTSD can last a lifetime due to observed and studied physical changes that occur in the brain following serious trauma.[2] This reason alone makes it vitally important to follow patients with this disorder and ensure that treatment is available.

Acute Stress Disorder (ASD) is a condition related to PTSD, but it is often overlooked. ASD usually emerges within two days to four weeks following a trauma, and most people who develop PTSD will have already developed ASD. ASD is a clinical reaction that occurs during the time prior to a patient developing and being diagnosed with PTSD. Depending upon which study is reviewed, anywhere from 50 percent to 80 percent of people with ASD will develop PTSD.[26] Although some wonder whether ASD is a milder form of PTSD and should be included with PTSD, the consensus is that ASD is not a minor variant of PTSD since there are significant diagnostic and treatment differences.

The diagnostic criteria for Acute Stress Disorder include:

1. Exposure to a trauma during which
   a. there was threatened death or serious injury, or a threat to physical integrity of self or others, and
   b. a response that involves intense fear, helplessness, or horror
2. Experiencing at least three of the following during or following trauma:
   a. Sense of numbing, detachment, or absence of emotional responsiveness
   b. A reduction in awareness of one's surroundings
   c. Derealization
   d. Depersonalization
   e. Dissociative amnesia
3. Re-experiencing the traumatic event in at least one of the following: recurrent images, thoughts, dreams, illusions, flashbacks, or a sense of reliving the experience; or distress on exposure to reminders of the trauma
4. Marked avoidance of stimuli that arouse recollections of the trauma
5. Marked symptoms of anxiety or increased arousal
6. Significant clinical distress or impairment in an important aspect of the person's life
7. Disturbance lasts at least two days and a maximum of four weeks and occurs within four weeks of the trauma
8. Reaction is not attributed to the effects of a substance or general medical condition or is not a brief psychotic episode or an exacerbation of another Axis I or Axis II disorder

Some question the validity of adding dissociative symptoms to the diagnostic criteria for ASD because there are multiple pathways to PTSD; that is, there are many different ways in which people can contract PTSD, although most people with ASD who do not have dissociative symptoms will go on to develop PTSD.[27] One does not have to experience dissociative symptoms to be diagnosed with either ASD or PTSD, although most clinicians think that dissociative symptoms should remain part of the diagnostic criteria since most people with Dissociative Disorders have experienced some type of trauma. If symptoms last longer than four weeks, then the person is suffering from an illness other than ASD. It may be PTSD, but it could be something else depending upon the symptom presentation. Not much is known at present about ASD, since people do not seek treatment unless their symptoms become worse. However, following an event such as rape and assault, the clinical picture of acute ASD is found in 70 percent to 90 percent of victims. The number who experience dissociative symptoms is not known, although one study showed that those who had been exposed to a firestorm reported a very high incidence of dissociative symptoms.[28]

Although we do not have a clear picture of who is likely to develop ASD, we find similarities with those who develop PTSD. People who experience more severe trauma, have preexisting psychopathology, have family and genetic vulnerability, have an abnormal personality, lack social support, and experience physical injury are more likely to develop ASD. In terms of differential diagnosis, a number of criteria must be considered. If psychotic symptoms are present, then the reaction to the trauma may be a brief Psychotic Disorder, the development of Major Depression, or both. If the ASD symptoms are the result of a physical injury, then the physical condition is probably the most appropriate diagnosis.

The course of ASD has not been well established, although Koopman et al.[28] found that the dissociative and cognitive symptoms that are common in ASD patients improve spontaneously over time in most cases. They also reported that the development of PTSD was more common among ASD patients with dissociative symptoms than among those with only anxiety symptoms; although, as mentioned above, some still question the inclusion of dissociative symptoms in diagnostic criteria for ASD.[29]

While ASD typically requires only the passage of time or minimal treatment or support to remit, the treatment picture for PTSD is usually different, although most victims of trauma do not develop PTSD and will return to normal functioning within a period of time. This finding supports the diathesis-stress model, which suggests that in order to develop PTSD a person must experience a traumatic event along with possessing some personal predisposing conditions; otherwise, everyone who experienced trauma would develop PTSD, and that is not the case. The high levels of comorbidity and symptom similarity between PTSD and Depression and Anxiety Disorders suggest that the same predisposing factors for these disorders are probably operative in PTSD patients as well.[30] There is evidence of some physiological, neuroanatomical, and neurophysiological differences in the bodies of people suffering from PTSD, but many findings are not clear about whether these were preexisting conditions that might have been vulnerability factors or if they were the result of changes in the body in response to significant trauma and stress.[31, 32, 33, 34, 35]

Additional factors may affect the development of PTSD, such as simple conditioning, which can explain why certain stimuli become related to the experience of trauma and then lead to similar feelings later. This relationship can also be important for treatment options. Solomon et al.[36] found that behavioral treatments using exposure to stimuli associated with fear or discomfort following the trauma could be helpful in treating PTSD. Scant but consistent evidence also shows that social support can be helpful to those suffering from PTSD, especially when the trauma involves the loss of a significant primary support system. It appears that social support is a buffer that helps to mitigate the effects of trauma, but the lack of social support places someone at additional risk for PTSD. Another risk factor for PTSD is the presence of Anxiety or Depressive Disorders among family members.[37] Evidence suggests that the psychiatric history of the person or of family members can influence two risk factors: first, it increases the likelihood of being exposed to a trauma; and, second, it increases the risk of developing PTSD once the person experiences trauma.[38]

A person who is exposed to trauma is at higher risk for several psychiatric illnesses, including Depression, some Anxiety Disorders, and PTSD, and treatment depends primarily on the types of symptoms presented and in what order. In addition to medical treatments (specific medications for specific symptoms), a number of psychological approaches are offered, including cognitive-behavioral therapy and exposure therapy, anxiety management training, and cognitive therapy.[39] Lundin provides some guidelines for the administration of treatment following a trauma:

- Brevity (keep it short and to the point)
- Immediacy (administer treatment soon after the trauma, if possible)
- Centrality (deal with issues central to the trauma)
- Expectancy (meet and explore the person's expectations for treatment)
- Proximity (treat the person close to the site of trauma, if possible)
- Simplicity (keep the treatment simple, straightforward)[40]

Civilian trauma survivors who developed ASD resorted to cognitive strategies of self-punishment and worry more so than survivors without ASD,[41] and treating survivors with cognitive-behavioral therapy has reduced these strategies and has increased the use of reappraisal and social control strategies.[2] The people who are at highest risk for traumatic stress disorders and who should be identified for treatment first include:

- Survivors with a psychiatric disorder
- Traumatically bereaved people
- Children, especially when separated from parents
- Individuals who are particularly dependent on psychosocial supports
  - Elderly
  - Handicapped
  - Mentally retarded
- Traumatized survivors
- Body handlers[2]

Although evidence shows that some people are more likely to benefit from treatment following trauma, there is no evidence to suggest that all survivors of trauma should be treated—screened, perhaps, but not necessarily treated. In fact, critical incident stress debriefing group sessions did not reduce the risk of developing PTSD later, and sometimes it seemed to worsen the symptoms. It appears that the best strategy is to first allow people to settle into their own coping styles and then offer treatment to those who do not improve.[42]

One type of individual who should be typically targeted for treatment following trauma is a person with a history of aggression, since PTSD is one path to increasing aggressiveness. In returning war veterans, there have been concerns regarding the increased possibility of intimate partner violence once back at home. To determine who is at higher risk for domestic or intimate partner violence, it is important to determine how much and what is perceived as a threat in the domestic environment.[43] Although treatments that are used for typical PTSD patients are also helpful in dealing with violent tendencies in PTSD patients, some interesting research has involved Conjoint Treatment for PTSD patients and their partners. This type of treatment involves:

- Psychoeducation to help the patient and his partner understand how PTSD affects their relationship
- Training in behavioral skills that improves listening and paraphrasing, assertiveness, and communication; the couple is taught to express emotions and to externalize and analyze their thoughts
- Taking newly learned skills and using them to improve communication and their relationship and to develop more trust and security

OBSESSIVE-COMPULSIVE DISORDER

Obsessive-Compulsive Disorder is frequently talked about, joked about, and written about, and many people believe they suffer from it or know someone who does. Persons with OCD typically experience persistent, upsetting thoughts and rituals that they use to control their anxiety, but, conversely, it is the rituals and the thoughts that end up controlling a significant part of a person's life. Obsessions are uncontrollable unwanted thoughts that make a person uncomfortable and force her to do something to keep the thoughts and anxiety at bay. Remember that we discussed the role of control in Anxiety Disorders in general? Obsession is another example of how the control issue is fundament to the disorder. People cannot control their thoughts and anxiety (obsessive part), so they engage in rituals that give them a sense of managing (controlling) them (compulsive part). Compulsions may include rituals such as checking, counting, performing specific tasks in a specific order, and touching things, but even if these behaviors temporarily relieve the anxiety, it always returns. These rituals are almost like strong superstitions; the person is usually aware that the rituals are irrational but fears that not performing them will result in something terrible happening.

Many people have obsessions or even exhibit compulsive behavior patterns, but that does not mean they have OCD. To qualify for an OCD diagnosis, behavioral patterns have to occur over a long period of time (e.g., months or years) and intrude into a person's life—a person with OCD may have good or bad days but the symptoms are always present. Obsessions and compulsions can also accompany other psychological disorders, for example, Obsessive-Compulsive Personality Disorder (OCPD). A person with this disorder has learned to live with obsessions and compulsions as habits more than symptoms. They are not as intrusive as the same symptoms of OCD, and OCPD lacks an anxiety component. These people experience obsessions without anxiety and become annoyed, perhaps, but not anxious; if prevented from fulfilling their compulsions, they still do not become anxious. Obsessions and compulsions are found in other Anxiety Disorders, such as Panic Disorder and Generalized Anxiety Disorder, but they are not as deeply ingrained nor as intrusive as they are in OCD.

Most adults with OCD know their ideas and behaviors are senseless; they say they feel crazy and try to hide their behaviors from others, often very creatively. However, some adult patients and most children with OCD feel that their behavior is perfectly reasonable and understandable, and these patients are diagnosed as having OCD with Poor Insight. It is estimated that OCD affects about 2.2 million American adults, many of whom live with comorbid conditions that further complicate their problems. Patients with OCD frequently suffer from Eating Disorders, other Anxiety Disorders, or Depression, and some self-medicate with alcohol or drugs. Men and women usually have similar rates of OCD (unlike most other Anxiety Disorders), and the condition usually emerges in childhood, adolescence, or young adulthood. Some evidence points to a genetic link in this disorder, but even if this is true, genetics alone is not enough to explain the full range of OCD symptoms.

OCD can be relatively mild or quite severe, and effective treatments usually include both medication and psychotherapy; one without the other is not as likely to be successful.[4]

The diagnostic criteria used by the American Psychiatric Association *DSM-IV-TR* include[18]:

1. Either obsessions or compulsions
   a. Obsessions defined by:
      i. Recurrent and persistent thoughts, impulses, or images that are typically experienced as intrusive and inappropriate and cause marked anxiety or distress
      ii. Not simply excessive worrying about real problems
      iii. Attempting to ignore or suppress such recurrent thoughts, impulses, or images, or to neutralize them with other thoughts or actions
      iv. Recognizing that recurrent thoughts are a product of one's own mind and are not imposed or inserted by outside agencies/people
   b. Compulsions defined by:
      i. Repetitive behaviors or mental acts that are aimed at preventing or reducing distress or preventing some dreaded event or situation; however, these are either not connected in a realistic way or are clearly excessive
2. At some point the person has recognized that the obsessions or compulsions are excessive or unreasonable, although this does not apply to children.
3. Obsessions or compulsions cause marked distress, are time consuming, and interfere with the normal aspects of a person's life.
4. If another Axis I Disorder is present, the content of the obsessions or compulsions is not restricted to it.
5. Disturbance is not due to the direct physiological effect of a substance (drug of abuse or medication) or a general medical condition.
6. Whoever is making the diagnosis of OCD must specify if the disorder is with poor insight.

OCD exists in all cultures and has been described in a variety of ways throughout history. It also appears that the basic types of obsessions and compulsions are consistent across cultures.[44] The most common types of obsessions are:

1. Fear of contamination (dirt and germs)
2. Pathological doubt
3. Need for symmetry
4. Aggressive obsessions[4]
5. Other obsessions
   a. Sexual
   b. Hoarding or collecting
   c. Religious
   d. Need to know something or remember things

    e. Fear of saying certain things
    f. Fear of not saying the right thing
    g. Intrusive (but neutral) images
    h. Intrusive nonsense sounds, words, or music
    i. Somatic

The most common compulsions are:

1. Checking
2. Washing
3. Symmetry
4. Need to ask or confess
5. Counting[2]
6. Some other compulsions that are seen:
    a. Repeating rituals
    b. Ordering or arranging
    c. Mental rituals other than counting or checking
    d. Touching certain things
    e. Measures to prevent causing harm to self, others, or things

Among children, most symptoms are similar, although washing compulsions followed by repeating rituals are the most common.[45] Most people with OCD have multiple obsessions and compulsions over time, with a particular fear or concern dominating at any given time, and the presence of obsessions without compulsions or vice versa is unusual.[2]

OCD may exist comorbidly and especially with Depression, which may predate the OCD or be caused by the complications of dealing with the OCD. In addition, OCD and other disorders can worsen during Depression. For example, one patient who had preexisting OCD was able to work and lead a normal life. However, he suffered a traumatic event at work and developed PTSD. Without question, the PTSD significantly impacted the OCD, worsening the OCD symptoms. The workers' compensation insurer tried to argue that his condition was preexisting and, therefore, not covered. The facts showed that the PTSD had its own symptoms that were causing new problems. The new PTSD condition had exacerbated the preexisting condition to the point where the man could not work. The court agreed, and he qualified for workers' compensation and ultimately for disability retirement.

Many believe there is frequent comorbidity with OCD and Tourette's syndrome or other Tic Disorders, but the relationship is not clear. Some report about a 5 percent to 10 percent comorbidity rate with OCD and Tourette's and 20 percent with other tics.[46] In addition, approximately 30 percent to 40 percent of people who already have Tourette's have high probability of developing OCD. In patients with Tourette's or other Tic Disorders, there is a greater probability of developing childhood-onset OCD and also more severe OCD symptoms.[47] Another disorder that is sometimes comorbid with OCD is Schizophrenia; patients who suffer from Schizophrenia or Schizoaffective Disorder have rates of OCD ranging from 8 percent to 46 percent, depending on the study.[48]

Until the mid-1980s, OCD was considered a rare disorder,[2] but the Epidemiologic Catchment Area Study[49] found OCD to be the fourth most common mental disorder, with a lifetime prevalence rate of 2.5 percent. The reported age of onset is usually during late adolescence. People who suffer from OCD will often report remembering problems in their childhood, although they covered them up or were dismissed and ignored by others. The earlier age of onset has been associated with an increased rate of OCD in first-degree relatives,[50] suggesting a familial type of OCD characterized by early onset, which usually means a worsening course.

Swedo et al. have described a type of OCD that begins before puberty and is characterized by an episodic course with intense exacerbations.[45] This has been linked with Group A beta-hemolytic streptococcal infections, which has led to the subtype designation of Pediatric Autoimmune Neuropsychiatric Disorders Associated with Streptococcal infections (PANDAS). In this study, the average age of onset was 7.4 years. Since this has only recently been identified, it is not yet clear whether this will be labeled a chronic condition with exacerbations. In more typical forms of OCD, the course tends to be characterized by waxing and waning severity, depending upon a number of factors, but a purely deteriorating or episodic course is not typical.[44]

In terms of differential diagnosis with OCD, there are a number of considerations. First, as mentioned above, obsessions and compulsions can occur with many other disorders besides OCD. To qualify for a diagnosis of OCD, the obsessions cannot be limited to the focus of another disorder, such as Body Dysmorphic Disorder or an Eating Disorder. However, if obsessions or compulsions are preoccupying as well as distressing or impairing, then it is probably OCD. As with other Anxiety Disorders, OCD uses avoidance to manage anxiety, but it also includes compulsions, which are not common to other Anxiety Disorders. As many as 60 percent of people with OCD also experience panic attacks, but unlike PD, these attacks only occur with exposure to a feared object or situation (e.g., dirt or contamination). Some Psychotic Disorders have obsessive features, but they rarely have the compulsive component, and Schizophrenia exhibits other symptoms such as hallucinations and thought disorders. Although OCD is not a Delusional Disorder, some types of delusions (e.g., somatic, jealousy) may be difficult to differentiate from OCD. However, these disorders will not usually have the anxiety component to the same extent.[2]

Some people confuse Impulse Control Disorders with OCD, since both disorders involve obsessing over what the person wants to do and the person may seem compulsive about her inability to control the behavior. But these two disorders are not the same, and Impulse Control Disorders will not present the other features of OCD. Therefore, if someone has kleptomania, trichotillomania, pathological gambling, sexual compulsions, and so forth, this is not the same as having OCD. With Impulse Control Disorders people enjoy or at least want to perform the act in question; OCD compulsions are not gratifying, although they may temporarily decrease anxiety. Fear and anxiety drive the compulsions in OCD, but this is not true in Impulse Control Disorders. Finally, some of the complex motor tics in Tourette's syndrome may be difficult to distinguish from OCD, but OCD is usually preceded by both anxiety and obsessional concerns, which is not true of Tourette's.[2]

Issues of etiology are complex and sometimes confusing in OCD. Some studies find structural and functional abnormalities in the brains of OCD patients.[51] Other neurobiological studies suggest an abnormality in the serotonin system,[52] and all of the antidepressants that effectively treat OCD affect serotonin levels.[53] Although the evidence of a role for the serotonin system in OCD is compelling, the actual role of serotonin in this disorder is not entirely clear. In some forms of OCD, especially with Tourette's, the balance of serotonin and dopamine systems may be important, and in that case, dopamine antagonists (neuroleptic medications) may improve therapeutic response.[2]

There is support for a genetic aspect of OCD, and in monozygotic twins a 63 percent concordance rate is very compelling evidence. However, since the concordance is not 100 percent, there must be environmental factors at work as well.[54] Pauls et al. studied first-degree relatives of OCD patients and 10.3 percent of them had OCD, 7.9 percent had subthreshold OCD, and these were significantly higher than for the control groups (1.9 percent for OCD, and 2 percent for subthreshold).[55] Pauls et al.[56] also reported higher rates of OCD in studies of families of people with Tourette's, and, conversely, Leonard et al.[46] found higher rates of Tourette's in the family members of someone who had OCD. Although ample evidence points to a role for genetics in OCD, it is unlikely that this disorder is a simple genetic disease.[57] Clearly, there is a role for the environment in the etiology of OCD as well.

A variety of psychological factors have been proposed for the understanding and treatment of OCD, but in recent years most of the attention has focused on learning approaches, with cognitive and behavioral perspectives predominating. Baer and Minichiello have presented a conditioning model for OCD that involves the negative reinforcement of compulsions.[58] This means that, to the extent that compulsions can reduce anxiety in the absence of confronting the feared stimulus, the compulsions are reinforced and more likely to continue; since the feared stimulus is not confronted, then extinction (elimination of anxiety) will not occur. The conditioning model for OCD is shown in Figure 6.1.

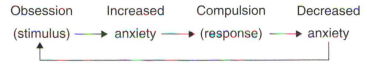

Figure 6.1 A Stimulus-Response Learning Model of OCD

Recent theory has attempted to integrate the biology of OCD with psychological models by proposing a phylogenetic model based on systems theory. In this model, behavioral inhibition and harm-assessment systems, which develop early in human phylogeny, are disrupted and can disrupt psychological processes, leading to psychological disorders. This can explain the diversity of symptoms seen in OCD.[59]

A number of effective treatment options are available involving psychopharmacologic and behavioral types of treatment in all age groups for OCD. Children and older adults seem to do very well with behavioral treatments and tolerate most of the medications, although at somewhat lower doses than adults. The goals of treatment for OCD patients are to reduce the frequency and intensity of symptoms as much as possible and to reduce or eliminate the amount of interference the symptoms have in the person's life. Typically, most patients do not experience a complete remission but can expect significant improvement with appropriate treatment. The most common course of the condition is a pattern of waxing and waning symptoms but not usually a total absence of symptoms.

7

Treatments for Anxiety Disorders

Do you want to know the surefire way to stay anxious? Don't do the thing
that makes you nervous!

—Latrina Kase, American author and psychologist

Treatments for Anxiety Disorders offer varying degrees of success, depending
on the accuracy and timeliness of the diagnosis, the type of treatment used,
the experience of the mental health professional, and the patient's personal
commitment to treatment. However, those who need treatment sometimes
do not receive it due primarily to a lack of awareness and poor access to treatment opportunities. Because many Anxiety Disorders are initially identified
at the primary care level, it is encouraging to note that in recent years physicians have become more aware of Anxiety Disorders and the basic types of
treatments available. When primary care providers, case management professionals, and providers of evidence-based psychotherapy and/or pharmacotherapy collaborate on the implementation of a treatment regime, patients
usually do very well.[1]

The primary goals of treatment involve reducing intrusive and troublesome
symptoms and controlling the need to avoid daily situations that consistently
threaten the patient with anticipated feelings of anxiety. Health care providers must also focus treatment efforts on decreasing the feelings of emotional
numbness that can accompany Anxiety Disorders and on helping patients
to stay actively involved in normal activities and to resist the temptation to
withdraw and become reclusive. Other treatment goals can involve dampen-
ing symptoms of hyperarousal and reducing impulse control problems when
necessary. Occasionally, Anxiety Disorders present with psychotic symptoms,
and these, too, must be addressed in treatment.

Additional treatment goals can help a patient learn to interpret events more realistically instead of exaggerating or inflating the risks they often infer from benign situations or things. Learning new and more appropriate responses and helping patients to improve their social functioning as well as their ability to relax and engage in leisure activities help a person feel more competent and in control and improves feelings of self-esteem, trust, and safety. Helping people to develop, utilize, and trust their support systems is also an important part of a comprehensive treatment plan, and, occasionally, there is a need to address historically important and intrusive issues emanating from a person's past. Ultimately, treatment involves assisting people to move from identifying themselves as victims to viewing themselves as survivors, and healthier because of their treatment.

Focusing on comorbid conditions is important in developing a comprehensive treatment plan. Often, patients enter treatment with multiple Anxiety diagnoses, Mood Disorders, Personality Disorders, or other problems. A common challenge in treating Anxiety Disorders involves dealing with the abuse of alcohol or other drugs. While these substances can temporarily ameliorate anxiety, alcohol and drugs often lead to addictions and serious complications that can make treatment and recovery even more difficult. While the problematic comorbidity between Anxiety Disorders and Substance Abuse is well known, there is much more to learn and more research is needed.[2]

In general, Anxiety Disorders are treated with medication, psychotherapy or both, depending on the patient's preferences and the approaches of the relevant treating professionals. Some patients begin treatment without mentioning to their therapist that they have previously tried and discontinued treatment in the past and are embarrassed for what they perceive as failure in the earlier efforts. It is important for those with Anxiety Disorders to understand that the "failures" are most often due to patients dropping out of treatment prematurely because they mistakenly believe that treatment is not working or, conversely, that they are cured. Many times the patient has simply not stayed with treatment long enough for it to be effective.

Medication is often the first type of treatment offered, because it produces the most immediate results and is usually the only type of treatment available at the primary care level. This can be either a positive or a negative step. While medication helps to reduce the symptoms of anxiety, it is rarely an adequate treatment by itself. When symptoms are under control, the patient can pursue psychotherapeutic types of treatment, which are more likely to produce effective and lasting results.[3] Specific types of drugs called *anxiolytic* or *antianxiety* drugs work well but often produce undesirable side effects that can hinder their use. Antidepressant medications are the most common drugs prescribed to treat Anxiety Disorders, and, and even if the patient does not suffer from Depression, these drugs reduce or control some of the symptoms of anxiety. Other types of drugs used to treat Anxiety Disorders include beta blockers, which may reduce anxiety but are usually used for treating high blood pressure, and antihistamines, which treat allergies and related disorders but can also lessen anxiety (they are also somewhat sedating). Occasionally, physicians will prescribe antipsychotic drugs for patients who are very agitated due to anxiety, but usually only for a limited time period. As discussed further on in this chapter, some alternative types of treatments are also occasionally used to treat Anxiety Disorders.

In addition to medication, psychotherapy has been successful in treating Anxiety Disorders, and there is considerable professional literature supporting its advances. The most recommended and thoroughly evaluated therapy is cognitive-behavioral therapy (CBT), which, together with medication, is most effective in treating Anxiety Disorders and in reducing disability from Anxiety Disorders, thus improving the quality of patients' lives. Although some medications work better with certain Anxiety Disorders, the cognitive-behavioral types of psychotherapy seem to work well for all types of Anxiety Disorders,[4] and some people are finding good results with newer forms of psychodynamic psychotherapy.[5]

Treatment for Anxiety Disorders does not always require medication, and some patients and providers prefer treatment without psychotropic drugs. Other helpful forms of psychotherapy and relaxation methods include biofeedback, where patients learn to use equipment that can help them to control physical responses related to anxiety. Other patients use yoga, meditation, and self-hypnosis.[3] A comprehensive treatment plan must include adequate sleep, moderate exercise, appropriate social activities, and proper nutrition, such as healthy eating and avoiding caffeine and alcohol.

MEDICAL TREATMENTS FOR ANXIETY DISORDERS

Medications are the most common medical treatments for Anxiety Disorders, with several successful drug strategies available and with proven efficacy. While the overall function of pharmacotherapy is to reduce symptoms to manageable levels so patients can return to a higher level of functioning and an improved quality of life, prescribing the appropriate drug(s) at the correct dosage is complex and challenging. Since not all primary care physicians (PCPs) are familiar with the numerous psychotropic medications and their side effects, and yet they are most often the first to diagnose and prescribe medical treatment for Anxiety Disorders, patients may not always receive the correct medication and dosage. Sometimes PCPs are reluctant to resort to *polypharmacy* (use of more than one drug) and are more likely to rely on a relatively limited range of medications. In addition, patients in some communities may have a limited number of psychiatrists or medically trained mental health professionals who can write prescriptions, and patients may face a lengthy waiting period for an appointment (sometimes three to six months). As the only available professional who can prescribe psychotropic medications, the PCP may delay referring patients to mental health professionals while they assess the effectiveness of the prescribed medication. This can result in a late referral, the delay of needed behavioral treatment, or in making any referral at all. Coordinated mental health care is also the responsibility of mental health professionals, who should maintain reasonable contact with PCPs regarding a mutual patient's treatment plan and make people aware of the services that they provide. As always, patients can be their own best advocate, inquiring about different types of treatment and requesting that their treating professionals stay in contact with one another.

Antidepressant Medications

The first line of medical treatment for Anxiety Disorders is usually selective serotonin reuptake inhibitors (SSRIs), which are relatively new drugs on the mental health scene. Although they were first used as antidepressants, they are also widely used for anxiety. They prevent serotonin from being absorbed back into the neuron that has discharged it, thus leaving more serotonin in the system to facilitate better transmission of the chemical messages between neurons in the brain. SSRIs are frequently used because they are generally well tolerated by most people and the side effects tend to be mild. Some patients experience nausea, which can be reduced by taking the drug with food; others may experience jitters, headaches, or sleep problems, and these side effects often diminish or disappear within a few days. If the side effects do not go away or are too uncomfortable to tolerate, the medication should be changed. Interestingly, if a person has side effects to one SSRI, that does not necessarily mean that he will have the same side effects with another SSRI. Occasionally, sexual side effects occur with the SSRIs, such as delayed orgasm, decreased sexual desire, or erectile dysfunction, and these may not disappear unless the dose or type of medication is changed. Some antidepressants are less likely to cause sexual side effects, and these might be used if the sexual side effects do not subside.

Another class of drugs called serotonin and norepinephrine reuptake inhibitors (SNRIs) inhibit the reuptake of both serotonin and norepinephrine. SNRIs tend to produce more side effects but can be helpful if the SSRIs are not effective in moderating anxiety. One specific SNRI, trazadone, produces the side effect of sedation and is often more helpful with insomnia than anxiety. Since trazadone is well tolerated in combination with SSRIs, it may be used when insomnia in an anxiety patient has worsened due to the use of an SSRI or if the patient's sleep problems were not improved by the SSRI.

Tricyclic antidepressants (TCAs) are also used to treat Anxiety Disorders, although not usually as a first-line treatment due to the side-effect profile. TCAs are an older class of drugs that have been in use for decades, but since the introduction of SSRIs, they are less frequently prescribed for Anxiety and Depression. Unlike the SSRIs, TCAs work with several neurotransmitter systems, but the treatment effect is not specific, and they tend to cause sedation, drying (e.g., mouth, eyes, nose), weight gain, and heart irregularities. Therefore, TCAs are rarely prescribed for older patients or anyone with a cardiac condition. Interestingly, they can be used in low doses to treat Chronic Pain Disorders and to prevent migraines, as well as to aid sleep in some patients. Unlike most of the TCAs, clomipramine works primarily on the serotonin system and is occasionally used for patients with Obsessive-Compulsive Disorder (OCD) but is rarely used with other anxiety conditions. A related tetracyclic called mirtazapine is beneficial in treating anxiety, is fairly sedating, and thus can be helpful with insomnia and particularly if taken at bedtime. However, it is rarely used as a first-line treatment due to undesirable side effects, including significant weight gain. Of course, not all patients will experience every side effect, but mirtazapine is not commonly used because there are other medications with fewer troublesome side effects, especially in the SSRI category.

The oldest class of antidepressants still used to treat Anxiety Disorders is the class of drugs called the monoamine oxidase inhibitors (MAOIs). These drugs are rarely used now in the United States but are more frequently prescribed in Europe and in other parts of the world. MAOIs have proven to be very effective in treating some types of Anxiety Disorders, especially Panic Disorder and Social Phobia. However, they can cause potentially serious side effects and are dangerous when taken with certain foods and with other medications. For example, MAOIs are possible sources of a dangerous interaction with some over-the-counter cold and cough medications. MAOIs are rarely used unless other available drugs have been deemed inappropriate, or nothing else has worked. A skin patch for an MAOI has been introduced and will probably prove to be much safer, but it has not been available for long and more research is needed.

Antianxiety (Anxiolytic) Medications

In addition to the antidepressant medications, another class of drugs that has been used to treat Anxiety Disorders for many decades is the antianxiety or anxiolytic medications, commonly known as tranquilizers. Until the last couple of decades, the main category of tranquilizers most often prescribed for the treatment of Anxiety Disorders was the benzodiazepines. Tranquilizers are generally quick acting and effective for anxiety—often taking effect within an hour or less. This differs significantly from most of the previously mentioned antidepressants, which may take a month or more to reach full effectiveness. Prior to the introduction of SSRIs, benzodiazepines were frequently used to treat anxiety, and at one point, Valium, a benzodiazepine, was the most frequently prescribed medication in the United States. Benzodiazepines work primarily by enhancing the production and availability of gamma-aminobutyric acid, which is a neurotransmitter related to controlling muscle tone, relaxation, and inhibition of excitatory processes.

As effective as tranquilizers can be, they are less frequently prescribed today, because they are addictive if taken for a long period of time and at a high enough dose. Also, increased tolerance can become an issue, which means a patient needs to continually increase the dosage for it to be effective. Tranquilizers also cause mild cognitive changes and drowsiness, a concern particularly for the elderly due to the increased risk of falling. People who take tranquilizers should know that there are 26 percent more motor vehicle accidents when people are taking benzodiazepines,[3] and these drugs are very dangerous when used with other drugs such as alcohol. Since tranquilizers work quickly, they are sometimes used as an adjunctive treatment with an SSRI, and as the SSRI becomes more effective over time, the benzodiazepine is tapered off.[6] Tranquilizers can also be useful for insomnia, as a muscle relaxant for many types of injuries, and for patients who are withdrawing from alcohol. Due to the addictive properties of tranquilizers, it is important for patients who are planning to discontinue a benzodiazepine to do so gradually and under the supervision of their physician or prescribing professional.

The anxiolytic drug buspirone is a safe drug with mild side effects that is nonaddicting and nonsedating. However, as a mild-acting drug, it is typically not very effective for moderate to severe anxiety problems. It can be used, however, for mild anxiety particularly if transient in nature. Another class of antianxiety drugs is the beta blockers. As mentioned earlier, these are primarily used to treat high blood pressure, angina pectoris, and other cardiovascular issues. However, beta blockers tend to be mildly anxiolytic (anxiety reducing) and are often helpful with Specific Social Phobias, such as stage fright.

A summary of drug types and dosage range are listed in Table 7.1.

Additional Medications and Natural Substances

Other drugs have been used experimentally for the treatment of Anxiety Disorders. For example, ketamine hydrochloride, commonly used as a general anesthetic, has been used for nonconventional applications in Substance Abuse rehabilitation due to its psychedelic properties. Data suggest that ketamine can be successfully applied for treatment in other Psychiatric Disorders

Table 7.1
Drugs Used to Treat Anxiety Disorders

Drug Type	Generic Name	Brand Names	Average Daily Dosage
Benzodiazepines	Alprazolam	Niravam	1–4 mg
		Xanax	1–4 mg
	Chlorazepate	Gen-Xene	15–90 mg
		Tranxene-SD	15–90 mg
		TranxeneT-TAB	15–90 mg
	Chlordiazepoxide	Librium	15–100 mg
	Clonazepam	Klonopin	1–4 mg
			4–40 mg
	Diazepam	Valium	1–2 mg
	Estazolam	ProSom	15–30 mg
	Flurazepam	Dalmane	2–10 mg
	Lorazepam	Ativan	30–120 mg
	Oxazepam	Serax	7.5–15 mg
	Quazepam	Doral	7.5–30 mg
	Temazepam	Restoril	0.125–0.25 mg
	Triazolam	Halcion	
Selective Serotonin Reuptake Inhibitors (SSRIs)	Citalopram	Celexa	20–40 mg
	Escitalopram	Lexapro	10–20 mg
	Fluoxetine	Prozac	40–60 mg
	Fluvoxamine	Luvox	50–300 mg
	Paroxetine	Paxil	20–50 mg
	Paroxetine (controlled release)	Paxil, CR	12.3–62.5 mg
	Sertraline	Zoloft	50–200 mg
Serotonin and Norepinephrine Reuptake Inhibitors (SNRIs)	Trazadone	Deseryl	150–400 mg
	Venlafaxine	Effexor	150–375 mg
	Venlafaxine (extended release)	Effexor XR	150–375 mg
	Desvenlafaxine	Pristiq	50 mg
Tetracyclics	Mirtazapine	Remeron	15–45 mg
		Remeron SolTab	15–45 mg

(*Continued*)

Table 7.1
Drugs Used to Treat Anxiety Disorders (*Continued*)

Drug Type	Generic Name	Brand Names	Average Daily Dosage
Tricyclics	Clomipramine	Anafranil	75–250 mg
	Desipramine	Norpramin	100–200 mg
	Imipramine	Tofranil	75–200 mg
	Nortriptyline	Aventyl	75–150 mg
		Pamelor	75–150 mg
Other Anxiolytics	Buspirone	BuSpar	10–30 mg
Beta Blockers	Acebutolol	Sectral	400–1,200 mg
	Atenolol	Tenormin	50–100 mg
	Bisoprolol	Zebeta	2.5–20 mg
	Carvedilol	Coreg	20–80 mg
	Metoprolol	Lopressor	50–200 mg
		Toprol XL	25–400 mg
	Nadolol	Corgard	40–80 mg
	Nebivolol	Bystolic	5–40 mg
	Propranolol	Inderal LA	120–160 mg

including Posttraumatic Stress Disorder (PTSD), phobias, and OCD;[7] however, the data are a bit premature and incomplete at present.

Some people have tried herbs and other natural substances as treatments for Anxiety Disorders with some interesting anecdotal testimonies to their effectiveness. For example, although there is no scientific evidence that kava works, some attest to its value. Although it is marketed as a natural treatment for anxiety, the Food and Drug Administration (FDA) recently warned that kava may cause liver damage and that long-term use can lead to allergies, visual disturbances, difficulties maintaining balance, and other problems. The FDA also states that kava should not be used during pregnancy or while breast-feeding and should never be used concurrently with antidepressants.[3] Valerian root is another natural substance that is taken primarily for insomnia, and, while it is also marketed for anxiety, very little data attest to its effectiveness.[3] Some have tried St. John's wort for anxiety, although it is primarily used for Depression, and the evidence regarding its efficacy in treating anxiety is minimal at best.

Some people think that taking natural substances is better than taking manufactured drugs because they are cheaper and safer—a very misleading perspective. "Natural" does not necessarily mean beneficial or safe. There are many poisonous and dangerous plants growing naturally that can be used as medicine, but all of their biological effects when applied or ingested have yet to be identified. Use of natural substances to treat psychiatric conditions, including anxiety, is possibly dangerous, deadly, or irresponsible at best. First, herbal and alternative substances do not fall under the purview of the FDA, and there is no established scientific body that provides reliable research and credible sources for claims of effectiveness and safety. Sellers of these products, of course, claim otherwise and are placing people at risk. Without coordinated scientific efforts to examine and evaluate effectiveness, side effects, drug interactions with prescribed and other medications (medical and psychiatric), other natural substances, and foods, to name just a few, it is potentially dangerous to depend on alternative substances as treatment for a psychiatric condition. If a patient is interested in taking natural substances, I recommend strongly that she seek information and advice from her physician and from a licensed professional trained in the use of alternative treatments. This professional (e.g., psychiatrist, physician's assistant, nurse practitioner, some psychologists, some pharmacists) can advise the patient regarding the risks and potential benefits of the alternative treatment and will have information about side effects, potential drug interactions, and other complications to be aware of. Following the treatment options that are the result of decades of quality scientific research and good clinical practice and that are offered by a competent mental health professional or physician is the safest and best path to improved mental health.

Pregnancy and Medications

Taking antianxiety medications during pregnancy or while breast-feeding is an important issue women of child-bearing age must consider. A woman who is, or expects to become, pregnant needs to consult with her prescribing professional and her obstetrician/gynecologist or family practitioner—whoever is following the pregnancy. While many mothers may prefer not to take medication during pregnancy or breast-feeding due to potential risks to the baby, a woman with untreated mental health problems can be an even bigger risk to the baby and to herself. The physician and patient can weigh all of the medical factors along with the preferences of the mother and together make a decision about continuing treatment.

Research indicates that SSRIs taken during the first trimester only marginally increase the risk of heart defects and are generally considered safe to take during early pregnancy. However, SSRIs taken later in pregnancy or at time of delivery may cause temporary problems in about 25 percent of newborns (e.g., tremor, restlessness, mild respiratory problems, weak cry).

Tricyclic antidepressants do not seem to cause problems with newborns at all. Bupropion does not appear to increase the risk of congenital malformations, but if it is taken during the first trimester, it may increase the risk of miscarriage.[8]

Antianxiety drugs present concerns for pregnant (or potentially pregnant) mothers, because benzodiazepines may increase the risk of cleft lip and cleft palate, although studies have produced inconsistent findings. We do know that the benzodiazepines may lead to withdrawal symptoms and other problems for newborns, especially if taken late in pregnancy.[8] Again, if a woman is taking any of these medications, she should discuss them with her physician before getting pregnant or as soon as she suspects that she is pregnant.

Other Medical Forms of Treatment

Medication is the most widely used medical treatment for Anxiety Disorders. Other treatments are available but are rarely used, because the evidence supporting their effectiveness is sparse. However, some patients (with OCD, for example) do not find traditional treatments effective at all, and medical treatments such as electroconvulsive therapy, transcranial magnetic stimulation, neurosurgery, and deep brain stimulation are available options. These treatments will be discussed in more detail in chapter 8.

PSYCHOLOGICAL TREATMENTS OF ANXIETY DISORDERS

As far back as Sigmund Freud in the late 19th and early 20th centuries, professionals have attempted to employ purely psychotherapeutic methods, without any medications, to treat Anxiety Disorders. In fact Jean Charcot, a French psychopathologist (a specialist who studies abnormal psychology) with whom Freud studied, demonstrated that the symptoms of "hysteria" could be temporarily relieved with hypnosis, a clear indication that this disorder was not purely physical in nature and could be treated with nonmedical types of therapies. Today, the evidence is clear that medication, while helpful in treating Anxiety Disorders, is rarely a cure by itself.

The most recommended psychotherapy for Anxiety Disorders is cognitive-behavioral therapy, an evidence-based form of treatment that is used in treating a myriad of Anxiety Disorders, including OCD. A variety of CBT techniques can be tailored to the individual and his symptoms, as well as to different groups and ages and in many different settings. Randomized controlled trials have consistently shown CBT to significantly reduce symptoms in children and youths, with a typical study showing that about two-thirds of children treated with CBT for Anxiety will improve.[9] It is not a template therapy method where each patient and each disorder is treated in a predictable and specific way. Rather, CBT is an approach that relies on the use of many different techniques that are designed to deal with each unique situation and individual and focus primarily on the changing of particular behaviors, developing better strategies for managing troublesome situations, and learning how to think about, perceive, and interpret circumstances in ways that lead to a healthier adaptation to conditions that are producing the symptoms. Examples of CBT techniques are:

- Psychoeducation on the nature of fear and anxiety
- Learning how to self-monitor symptoms
- Relaxation and breathing retraining
- Cognitive restructuring (learning how to think differently about anxiety issues)
- Behavioral experiments (trying to do things differently)
- Imaginal and in vivo exposure to feared images, bodily sensations, and situations
- Learning to ignore or to not fixate on warning signs
- Response and relapse prevention techniques

CBT is not a quick fix, although some techniques are considered short-term oriented. Research suggests that a patient may not notice significant improvement with CBT for 12 weeks or more, which is why patients who are receiving CBT will also take medication and why patients sometimes terminate their own therapy too soon. It is important for patients to understand that the drugs will often produce a quick treatment response, but it is the CBT that will ultimately produce long-lasting results and reduce or eliminate the need for continued medication. CBT is appropriate and effective in individual psychotherapy or in group therapy settings,[10] but patients usually prefer individual over group therapy.[11] Although CBT offers robust treatment effects and has proven effective in a variety of settings and over extended follow-up periods, there is still much to learn about the prevention of Anxiety Disorders and the advantages of early intervention.[12]

CBT involves many interdependent factors that must be addressed in order to produce the desired behavioral changes and reach the goals established by the patient and the treating professional. Advocates of CBT believe that chronic negative thinking (cognitive factors) leads to feeling poorly, both physically and emotionally (emotional factors), which then leads people to do things (behavioral factors) that perpetuate or exacerbate the negative thinking and feelings. CBT teaches people how to break this cycle by changing how they act (behavior) and think (cognitive), which will then lead to feeling differently. Research support for CBT is very positive and indicates that patients going through CBT treatment, for any type of Anxiety Disorder, usually feel much better following treatment.

Cognitive techniques in CBT attempt to change the way people think about their problems and about the issues they face. A therapist helps the patient to recognize and view the situations or stimuli that produce anxiety and develop cognitive strategies for dealing with them in a more functional manner. Using cognitive rehearsal and imagining how to do things differently help a patient to initiate new behaviors. A technique called reframing is frequently employed to help people learn new ways to think about particular problems or situations.

In addition to cognitive strategies, CBT relies heavily on behavioral techniques, especially during the beginning phases of treatment. It is easier for patients to change how they act than how they think, and it is easier to change how they think than how they feel; so treatment begins by working to change the easiest things first—behavior. By helping people to behave differently in a situation where previously they were too anxious to act normally, they will begin to feel safe enough to try new behaviors. Using exposure methods also helps them to face situations that were previously very frightening, thereby gaining self-confidence and reducing the need to avoid the situations or stimuli that evoke their feelings of anxiety. For example, people with Generalized Anxiety Disorder worry continuously and tend to expect the worst-case scenario, which then causes them to act and feel as if the event has actually occurred.[11] Encouraging patients to approach situations where the worst-case scenario *does not* occur, helps them to feel more comfortable and safe and assigning homework to patients between appointments is also a frequent element of CBT.[11] Patients need to understand that a few hours per month of psychotherapy are not going to change entrenched behavioral patterns. Patients' efforts outside of the therapy office in their daily routines will determine how quickly they notice improvements. Use of exposure techniques in CBT means repeated and systematic confrontation of the feared stimuli but in a manner that is manageable and safe, stressing that the feared outcome does not actually occur—the anxiety then decreases or disappears. Exposure, or at least exposure-like principles, is the common theme in most of the new treatment methods, and most outcome studies are very favorable—clearly, these techniques frequently work well.[13] Although exposure is a major element of CBT, there is still much to discover about what it does and how it works.[14]

The use of CBT for Anxiety Disorders is the most effective and most accepted treatment according to available research and reports.[15] One set of studies did a meta-analysis of CBT studies and found that the results were equally effective in laboratory studies as in clinical settings and were effective with all of the Anxiety Disorders; across the board, CBT techniques have been described as highly effective.[16] Meta-analytic studies take all the data from an entire body of related experimental literature and then combine and analyze them in ways that allow broader conclusions to be drawn. One additional study by Stewart used meta-analytic techniques and found that CBT for Anxiety Disorders does successfully generalize to clinical practice settings and is effective in situations outside of the lab or structured clinical settings.[17] As effective and helpful as CBT appears to be for Anxiety Disorders, practitioners who are not well trained or who do not follow the accepted methods produce less impressive results.[15]

There are some variants of cognitive-behavioral therapy, as well as several types of therapy that are not CBT, and many of them use some of the same techniques. Most schools of therapy for anxiety realize that use of cognitive techniques must include an element of exposure to be effective.[18] For example, the treatment of PTSD involves a number of therapies, but the preponderance of evidence says that the primary effective component of PTSD treatment is prolonged exposure to troubling or anxiety-provoking stimuli or situations.[19] Many behavioral techniques such as relaxation training, meditation, mindfulness therapy, yoga, and biofeedback help people to manage their anxiety, which helps them to minimize the worry and resultant fears. The chosen approach to treatment often involves a strategy for targeting the most intrusive or troublesome symptoms first or, in some cases, for dealing with comorbid conditions before tackling anxiety issues. For example, if a person suffers from an Anxiety Disorder as well as a Substance Use Disorder, treating the anxiety while the person is still abusing the substance is counterproductive. It is often difficult to convince a patient of this fact due to the patient's limited understanding of anxiety and the mistaken assumption that eliminating the anxiety will also eliminate the need to drink or use drugs. However, the process actually works in reverse. The use of a substance negatively affects the anxiety, making the anxiety symptoms more difficult to treat, and the use of drugs or alcohol complicates the effectiveness of the medications prescribed and can be a danger in combination. Many of these techniques are used primarily with adults; they have not been thoroughly evaluated in the treatment of children and require more research in this area.

OTHER PSYCHOSOCIAL TREATMENT APPROACHES

One area of study in the cognitive treatment of Anxiety Disorders has focused on cognitive bias. This refers to the tendency of people with anxiety problems to perceive or think about certain things in a biased or exaggerated fashion—that is, to magnify the actual risk or probability of a given feared outcome. Although it has been demonstrated that anxious people will selectively attend to and interpret situations in ways that are consistent with their fears, the use of an approach called cognitive bias modification has been very successful in reducing symptoms of Anxiety and Depression and adapting to other forms of therapy.[20]

Relaxation training is another approach for treating Anxiety Disorders, although some have questioned the relative contribution of relaxation and specific cognitive approaches. Siev found that both relaxation therapy and cognitive approaches were effective in the treatment of general anxiety, anxiety-related cognitions, and Depression for patients with Generalized Anxiety Disorder.[21] However, for patients with Panic Disorder, either cognitive therapy or CBT produced the best results. Relaxation techniques are generally not used alone but are one element of a more comprehensive treatment.

While speculating as to why the behavioral techniques are so effective, some have posited that a *connection mechanism* is responsible for some of the behavioral methods being successful.[22] For example, placing a person in a situation where she is required to do something that she fears will result in feelings of *dissonance*, anxiety about doing something she really does not want to do. Therefore, there is a connection between what she is doing and the experience of anxiety. However, as behavioral techniques are continued in a safe manner, the person now experiences an *induction* of new connections, and the old, established connections between a given set of stimuli and fears are replaced by feelings of safety and comfort in a situation that had previously produced fear and anxiety.

CBT techniques have been so successful and well accepted that they are now integrated into other forms of therapy, such as family therapy.[23] Carr points out that experimental evidence supports the benefits of combining family therapy with other systematic approaches for the treatment of anxiety.[24] For example, a family with three young children began treatment for one of their children who was suffering from Anxiety Disorder. The therapist saw the child individually at first but also relied on parental counseling to help the parents understand the disorder and the methods of treatment. As the youngster improved, the therapist scheduled family therapy sessions to generalize the CBT techniques to the rest of the family and to more effectively help them deal with the situations that had been stressful for all of them. A different approach was studied in Sweden and in the United States that used a focused one-session treatment for Specific Phobias in anxious youths; it was very effective and demonstrated that the treatment effects were upheld even on follow-up.[25]

Some other creative clinicians have proposed combining a variety of techniques that can interface with the inclination of many teens to be heavily involved with technology. For example, Eagle suggests the use of mindfulness-informed and technology-incorporating techniques in group therapy for anxious adolescents.[26] Another technology-based form of treatment for anxiety is the application of Internet and computer-based therapy (ICT); the intent is to reduce the cost and improve the availability of treatment. In one meta-analytic study, ICT was better than wait list groups across all treatment measures, and ICT was as good as therapist-delivered treatment across different Anxiety Disorders. It must be pointed out that these studies involved small samples and no placebo controls. However, ICT was found to be a reasonable treatment for some Anxiety Disorders.[27]

Additional forms of treatment are psychodynamic therapies, and many maintain that these methods have been overlooked in the treatment of Anxiety Disorders and should be considered a mainline treatment. Psychodynamic therapists typically view the interpretation of the traumatic events that are associated with symptoms as being critical to determining the experience and impact of the Anxiety Disorders. Treatment is then geared toward altering attributions (the patient's assumed causes of the symptoms) by slow exposure and through confrontation and awareness of the negative emotions that have been generated by the trauma. This usually provokes certain troublesome conflicts that must be confronted. The key in this type of treatment is to keep the level of a patient's reactions to confrontations within tolerable limits. In the past, courses of sychodynamic therapies were typically quite long and not available to many patients, although some patients do well with these techniques. Proponents of this approach point out that, while CBT is proven to be effective, some patients do not respond well to it. Often, there are relapses when patients discontinue medication, and some do not like or cannot tolerate the behavioral techniques. Further, there is sparse evidence on the effects of CBT on problems such as occupational functioning, relationship difficulties, and diminished quality of life.[5]

A less frequently utilized treatment technique is hypnosis, which dates back to Charcot and Freud. Some use hypnosis today to desensitize patients to feared stimuli and situations or as a helpful tool in teaching relaxation techniques. However, a strong warning is offered: Hypnosis is not a legally licensed profession, and many who practice it are not adequately or professionally trained. Many hypnotists advertise memberships to official-sounding organizations with no legal or professional merit. If a patient wants to try hypnosis to help treat an Anxiety Disorder, the patient should find a licensed professional (e.g., psychologist, psychiatrist, or social worker) who is trained specifically in hypnosis. Since the research literature is not supportive of hypnosis as a primary treatment method for Anxiety Disorders, it is not an advocated technique. Some controlled research found that the use of hypnosis is no more effective than a placebo; however, it might occasionally be helpful in the hands of a competent professional who uses it as a part of a total treatment program.[28] Many people harbor serious misconceptions about the effectiveness of hypnosis and mistakenly think that being hypnotized a couple of times will force their anxiety to disappear—unfortunately, it is never that simple.

Eye movement desensitization and reprogramming (EMDR) therapy has attracted considerable attention in recent years, and especially in the treatment of PTSD. This approach relies on a variety of techniques that are supposed to treat the symptoms of Anxiety Disorders. In addition to PTSD, EMDR has been used to treat Phobias, Panic Disorder, grief, chemical dependency, and Dissociative Disorders. A major meta-analytic study by the Institute of Medicine (IOM) did not find that EMDR was an effective treatment for PTSD and that the effects, if any, were not strong. Although there are claims of the successful use of EMDR, most of the confirmatory results were based solely on self-report measures and anecdotal case studies. Physiological indices of the effects of trauma did not support the treatment claims. In fact, many studies reported that there was no evidence of therapeutic effect at all.[29] Some writers feel that the IOM meta-analysis was inadequate and unfair,[30] but other more confirmatory meta-analyses have not yet been issued; until additional studies are conducted, there is not enough evidence to oppose the IOM study.

Once again, if someone is interested in seeking EMDR treatment, he should locate a licensed treatment professional who offers it and discuss whether it may be helpful. Some reputable providers will use this technique as one element of a total treatment program but rarely as the sole modality of treatment. Further research and analysis are needed on approaches such as hypnosis and EMDR before they can be endorsed or rejected.

One new strategy that is gaining considerable attention and support is mindfulness meditation, an acceptance-based approach to dealing with psychological problems with a long history (e.g., Buddhist traditions and Rogers[31]). This approach incorporates some cognitive techniques with relaxation types of therapy and looks very promising.[28] What is particularly helpful is that this approach is easily incorporated into other treatment methods, including CBT as well as most other forms of psychotherapy, and is generating both interest and research.[32] Recent studies demonstrated that mindfulness meditation training can produce a significant reduction in Anxiety and Depression following treatment and that the number of patients who reported panic attacks also decreased. They also found that a mindfulness meditation training group can effectively reduce symptoms of anxiety and panic and can help maintain these reductions in patients with a variety of Anxiety Disorders.[33]

Some providers have focused more on the acceptance aspects of treatment, emphasizing the notion that commitment on the part of the patient is an important element when dealing with Anxiety Disorders. The approach is often referred to as acceptance and commitment therapy (ACT), and it is very similar to other mindfulness treatments. The research literature finds that ACT may be an effective treatment for a variety of disorders, including several Anxiety Disorders, Depression, pain, trichotillomania, Psychotic Disorders, drug abuse, and the management of epilepsy and diabetes. Evidence suggests, however, that ACT works through different processes than those involved in other forms of treatment, including traditional CBT;[34] however, some suggest that ACT and CBT are more alike than different.[35] Although newer mindfulness and ACT approaches are encouraging, more research and experience are necessary to determine how to effectively employ these techniques. Other therapists have used the basic approaches from positive psychology in the treatment of Anxiety Disorders, and results have been encouraging.[36] This approach focuses on positive, actively involved approaches to help people deal with their problems, and, as with mindfulness and ACT, this set of techniques helps to empower patients to be able to approach and deal with their difficulties in positive, proactive ways.

SUMMARY

The various cognitive and behavioral approaches to treatment seem to have much in common, and a combination of approaches may be helpful to an overall treatment plan. In addition, there is no evidence that combining treatments will compromise the efficacy of treatment in general.[37] Similarly, many researchers have studied the combination of medication and CBT and have concluded that it is the best and most comprehensive approach to treating Anxiety Disorders. However, the literature does not find that the outcome of CBT itself is improved by combining it with medication.[28] While this might seem to argue against the use of medication in the treatment of Anxiety Disorders, there are enough findings that demonstrate a useful role for medication in treatment for it not to be totally discounted. Therefore, if a patient is seeking treatment for anxiety problems and wants to avoid medication, there are several effective psychosocial treatments to use without medication. A promising approach used more frequently today takes advantage of the short-term benefits of medication, when appropriate, and couples it with the long-term benefits of psychosocial treatments. Many available and effective therapies can be combined to offer an encouraging variety of accepted and successful treatment methods that will help to improve patients' lives.

8

Treatment Methods for Specific Anxiety Disorders and Patient Groups

> In between attacks there is this dread and anxiety that it is going to happen again. I'm afraid to go back to places where I've had an attack. Unless I get help, there soon won't be anyplace where I can feel safe from panic.
> —Anonymous quote from National Institute of Mental Health,
> "Anxiety Disorders," www.nimh.nih.gov/health/publications/
> anxiety-disorders/complete-index.shtml

A variety of medical and psychotherapeutic treatment methods are available to patients who suffer from any of the types of Anxiety Disorders, but certain strategies are more effective than others when applied to specific disorders. Determining the correct course(s) of therapy can be complex and challenging to both the professional and the patient, and each unique client requires careful consideration prior to choosing the method(s) deemed most likely to be helpful. The following guidelines of treatment for specific Anxiety Disorders and suggested specific treatment methods summarizes the current research and is not intended to be the best approach for every patient.

PANIC DISORDER

Typically, the first line of treatment for Panic Disorder includes a combination of medication and psychotherapy—usually a selective serotonin reuptake inhibitor (SSRI) or a serotonin and norepinephrine reuptake inhibitor (SNRI) with cognitive-behavioral therapy (CBT)—and usually requires a longer term of treatment than for some of the other Anxiety Disorders. Since antidepressant medications are not fully effective for at least a month, the additional temporary use of a faster-acting benzodiazepine tranquilizer, such as alprazolam, can reduce symptoms of anxiety and panic in the short term and be tapered off when the antidepressant and psychotherapy produce a noticeable change.[1] While adding a tranquilizer can be helpful during early stages of treatment, it is usually not helpful during the later stages of psychotherapy. It is reported that 50 percent to 70 percent of patients with Panic Disorder respond to medication or psychotherapy during the first few months of treatment, and about 25 percent to 50 percent of patients, who discontinue taking medication (for whatever reason), suffer a relapse within six months. The International Cochrane Collaboration concluded that medication with psychotherapy or psychotherapy alone (never medication alone) should be the first treatment options offered to patients with Panic Disorder.[2] Because Panic Disorder is a chronic condition, the clinician and patient must first deal with the acute phase of the disorder, which includes the first few months when the panic attacks are coming under control, and then address the minimization and prevention of future attacks and the anticipatory anxiety that usually precedes them. It is vital that patients maintain a healthy lifestyle, including adequate sleep and rest, regular exercise, good nutrition, and cessation of nicotine and caffeine products, which often can precipitate panic attacks in patients with Panic Disorder. Some patients do not respond well to the suggested standard treatments, and providers can then apply alternate treatment modalities or can refer a patient to another professional who offers different methods.

GENERALIZED ANXIETY DISORDER

For many years providers have used the benzodiazepine tranquilizers as the first-line treatment for Generalized Anxiety Disorder (GAD).[3] However, today many consider their long-term use a serious concern due to the side effect profile.[4] In fact, in recent years the chronic use of these drugs for the treatment of GAD has been increasingly discouraged.[5] Alternatively, tricyclic antidepressants (TCAs) have been helpful in the treatment of GAD.[6] One study found that the tranquilizer diazepam was effective during the first two weeks of treatment but not more effective than a TCA later.[7] Most frequently, the SSRIs[3] and the SNRIs[8] are used as the first-line treatment for GAD. Buspirone has also been used to treat GAD, with mixed results, and is typically not used unless a patient does not tolerate the more commonly used medications. (Please see Table 7.1 for helpful descriptions of specific drugs.)

Although medications can be effective with GAD, they are not an adequate and effective treatment alone, since they usually lead to a relapse after their termination. Psychosocial treatments are vital elements of treating GAD, and most patients respond very well to the combination of medication and psychotherapy.[1] Of the psychosocial treatments, CBT is the most effective psychotherapeutic treatment in the research literature, although some patients with milder forms of GAD have progressed as a result of alternative types of treatment, including supportive therapy. Relaxation, alone or with other treatments,[1] plus a newer form of psychotherapy that is similar in many ways to CBT called acceptance-based behavior therapy have also proven effective for GAD patients.[9] In addition, the Attention Modification types of therapies can help people to change how they think about things and how they attend to them.[10]

SOCIAL ANXIETY DISORDER

People who suffer clinically relevant Social Anxiety Disorder, or Social Phobia—the fear of being negatively evaluated by others and the subsequent avoidance of social situations—often avoid treatment because they are afraid and embarrassed to deal with the issues related to this condition. Only about 5 percent of people with Social Phobia have sought mental health services, and only about 20 percent have been treated by a professional for an emotional problem of any type. Effective treatments for Social Phobia involve both medication, usually an SSRI or SNRI, and psychotherapy.[11]

A subtype of this disorder is known as Specific Social Disorder, which is a debilitating fear that produces symptoms only in specific situations (e.g., stage fright or fear of public speaking). People often respond well to a beta blocker if it is taken prior to entering a feared situation. Often, medication treatment alone is adequate until the client gains enough confidence to proceed without it. Beta blockers are used primarily for treating high blood pressure but can be effective for some mild anxiety conditions.

Treatment for General or Specific Social Phobias usually involves the CBT method of psychotherapy, as well as social skills training and/or exposure and desensitization. One consideration in the treatment of Social Phobia is whether there is a comorbid condition. For example, people with Social Phobia are more likely to suffer from Depression and Substance Abuse, and if either or both of these are present, these disorders must be treated as well.[12]

When treating any type of Phobia, simply discussing with a patient those things or situations that cause anxiety will typically produce anxious feelings during the conversation. The treating professional must, therefore, conduct the discussion in a manner that does not escalate the anxiety to an intolerable level or create a therapeutic environment that the patient would want to avoid.

Early identification and treatment is important when treating Social Phobia in order to prevent the development of a chronic course of symptoms, persistent functional impairment, and progressive psychiatric comorbidity. Fortunately, effective treatments are available to all age groups. Emerging literature supports the use of CBT for Social Phobia in youths, and one study showed that CBT and educational/supportive psychotherapy were both effective in treating Social Phobia in teens, but CBT showed greater gains on the behavioral measures.[13]

Although the efficacy of CBT for Social Phobia is well established, it is a complex set of procedures, not just a list of techniques, and it is not yet clear which elements of the therapeutic method are the most effective or why. Studies have also established that the cognitive techniques, as well as relaxation and exposure methods, are helpful in treating Social Phobia, making it apparent that these parts of the total treatment approach are important.[14] Another study demonstrated that individual treatments for Social Phobia may be superior to group therapy regardless of the treatment type.[15]

SPECIFIC PHOBIA

The main goal when treating Phobias is to decrease the fear and phobic avoidance to a level that no longer causes significant distress or functional impairment.[16] Specific Phobia requires a slightly different approach because it involves a particular situation or object that evokes fear, and the treatment will depend on a variety of considerations, including how often the person confronts the feared object or situation. Although it is common to treat Specific Phobias with both medication and psychotherapy, the choice of medication also depends on factors such as frequency of exposure. For example, if a person suffers from a fear of flying but only flies a few times a year, it is not necessary for her to take daily medication.

A patient was referred to me with a severe fear of flying, and he reported that he needed to fly each month for his job. Collaborating with his physician, I suggested a combination of alprazolam, a benzodiazepine tranquilizer that works fast and then wears off quickly, and CBT to treat him. As he progressed, the physician reduced the dose of alprazolam for each flight until the patient did not need any medication when he flew; once he was relatively free of anxiety when he flew, I discharged him from treatment. I saw him about a year later in a social situation, where he mentioned that he had not used the alprazolam since he last saw me. However, he confessed in a somewhat embarrassed manner that he always made sure that he had at least one tablet in his pocket whenever he flew. "Isn't that kind of crazy, Doc?" he asked me. I assured him that not only was it *not* crazy, it was a good security blanket if it made flying easier. I ran into him again several months later, and he had a big smile on his face when he said, "You knew what would happen, didn't you?" I laughed and said, "You forgot to take the alprazolam with you!" At the moment he discovered that he had, indeed, forgotten to put the pills in his pocket, he had started to laugh because it was then he realized that the medication no longer had anything to do with his ability to fly. The point of this example is to stress that, when designing a treatment program, providers must make decisions regarding treatment that depend upon the type of Phobia presented, how and when it is problematic, the specific symptoms involved, and the severity of the symptoms.

Although medication is an appropriate strategy for some situations, daily medication alone is not a long-term solution, since once the drug is discontinued, the symptoms will return. Also, if a person has a Phobia about something she will never experience (e.g., an intense fear of being swallowed by a huge snake), treatment is only warranted if the Phobia actually interferes with the person's life. Therefore, if the person is content to avoid those parts of the world where huge snakes exist, the Phobia is not a problem and treatment is not necessary.

Specific Phobias respond most often to psychotherapy, with CBT providing good, long-term results and rare relapses. The most effective element of CBT seems to be exposure, where the patient experiences the feared stimulus, sometimes repeatedly, under controlled conditions (sometimes in vivo [in real life] and sometimes imaginal); then, the person gradually learns to face the stimulus without becoming anxious. Findings from research literature on exposure include:

- Exposure seems to work best when sessions are spaced close together.
- Prolonged exposure seems to be more effective than exposure of shorter durations.
- During exposure sessions, individuals should be discouraged from engaging in subtle avoidance strategies, like distracting themselves.
- Real-life exposure appears to be more effective than exposure through imagination.
- Exposure with therapist involvement seems to be more effective than exposure conducted without a therapist present.
- Exposure can be gradual or abrupt and both are effective, although patients usually prefer the more gradual methods.
- In Blood and Injection Phobias, the technique of applied muscle tension (to increase blood pressure) is effective with exposure,[16] as this will prevent or minimize the chance of the person fainting.

Research and practice demonstrate decisively that Simple Phobias are among the most treatable of all the Anxiety Disorders[16] and that those who suffer from them should be referred as soon as possible to a mental health professional that specializes in the treatment of Phobias. New methods of CBT that take advantage of technologies such as computers, videos, and other electronics can also help people to deal with these types of issues.[16]

OBSESSIVE-COMPULSIVE DISORDER

Generally, a combination treatment of CBT and medication is the approach taken with Obsessive-Compulsive Disorder (OCD). The SSRIs are the first line of treatment, and the second line is often another SSRI or clomipramine, which is seldom used as a first-line treatment due to its undesirable side effect profile. There is no evidence that one SSRI is superior to the others; all of them have demonstrated efficacy.[17] However, some patients will respond better to one over another, although it is often difficult to determine which one will work the best without trying it. Looking only at SSRIs, 40 percent to 60 percent of patients showed symptom reduction, although most continued to report residual symptoms.[17] OCD seems to require higher dosages of the SSRIs than does Depression, and, while some improvement in depressive symptoms is usually seen within 2 to 6 weeks of pharmacotherapy, it may take 10 to 12 weeks to see an improvement of OCD symptoms. One challenge to using medication for OCD is that patients often relapse when drugs are terminated, and some providers find that individual patients may require continued medication indefinitely. However, when medication is combined with CBT, relapse rates are much lower.

A course of treatment for OCD is never a quick fix, and before a provider decides to change the mode of treatment due to a lack of perceived progress, the patient should take medication for at least 10 to 12 weeks and/or participate in 13 to 20 weeks of CBT.[17] If the SSRIs are not producing the desired effect, there are other medications or augmentation options, where a second medication is added, such as antipsychotic drugs, to the SSRI or any other primary drug. In fact, 40 percent to 55 percent of patients who have not responded to an SSRI will improve with an antipsychotic. Clomipramine can be used as an augmentation agent to an SSRI. Because clomipramine can cause arrhythmias and even death in people with heart problems, it should not be used with anyone over the age of 40 or with a history of cardiac disease.[16] Also, clomipramine should not be used with fluvoxamine, fluoxetine, or paroxetine, because these drugs will increase the blood levels of clomipramine to a troublesome degree.[17] Some recent studies have shown that intravenous clomipramine acts quicker with fewer side effects than the oral medication and may be effective for people who did not respond to the oral form. Koran et al. showed a therapeutic response in four and a half days when using an intravenous pulse dosing of clomipramine.[18]

If augmentation of SSRIs is not effective, the next step is to change medications. Research has established that 50 percent of patients who do not respond to one SSRI will respond to a different one.[17] Current clinical practice suggests that, if there is no response to an SSRI, it is best to change to another SSRI, but if there has been a partial response, then using an augmentation trial may be warranted.[19, 20] Another study on a specific medication strategy reported that patients with OCD who also suffered from symptoms of compulsive hoarding seemed to respond well to paroxetine.[1]

Although medication is often the first line of treatment, considerable evidence indicates that medication alone is not adequate treatment for OCD and that psychosocial treatment is an important part of the treatment regime. Of the various psychotherapies, CBT is the most studied in the treatment of OCD, and its robust treatment effects have been established across a variety of treatment settings and over extended periods of time.[21] The behavioral forms of treatment have also been established both as an effective primary treatment and as an augmentation agent when used with medication.[22] The techniques usually employed when working with OCD patients are exposure to the things and situations that patients obsessively worry about (e.g., germs) and response prevention, when the person is prevented from completing his compulsive rituals. The exposure can be in vivo or imagined,[23] although many feel that the in vivo treatment is more effective. Of course, other behavioral treatments can be used, depending upon the individual patient and her symptoms.

Research shows that 50 percent to 70 percent of patients respond to behavioral treatment alone, which is especially helpful for patients with Contamination or Somatization Fears that cause them to want to avoid medication.[16] Some have asserted that combination therapy—behavioral and medication—is the best for OCD patients, but this is still a preliminary conclusion.[24] Others have demonstrated that adding pharmacotherapy to behavioral treatment may be helpful in reducing obsessions, while compulsions respond better to behavior therapy.[25] The most common form of OCD treatment begins with medication, followed by the addition of behavioral therapy as the patient becomes more comfortable with treatment. O'Sullivan and Marks found that in one to six follow-ups, 75 percent of patients treated with behavior therapy continued to do well, although few were completely symptom free.[26] Psychoanalytic and supportive psychotherapy have not proven helpful with OCD, although they may be more effective with Obsessive-Compulsive Personality Disorder,[16] which is similar to OCD but is not categorized as an Anxiety Disorder.

As effective as CBT has proven to be with patients who have OCD, 15 percent to 25 percent of patients refuse initially to engage in behavioral treatment or discontinue treatment early because it is too anxiety-provoking for them. Another 25 percent drop out for other reasons, such as comorbid Depression; lack of insight; use of central nervous system depressants, which may lessen anxiety and motivation for treatment; poor compliance with treatment; or poor compliance of the therapist with accepted treatment methods.[22]

Roughly 10 percent of patients with OCD will worsen despite treatment and may be candidates for other forms of medical treatment. Patients who do not improve despite multiple medication trials in addition to CBT may be candidates for brain surgery or deep brain stimulation. Some have tried electroconvulsive therapy and transcranial magnetic stimulation for the treatment of OCD, but these have not proven to be effective.[16] Most surgical techniques for OCD rely upon ablation (the destruction of tissue) and include:

- Anterior capsulotomy
- Limbic leucotomy
- Cingulotomy
- Gamma-knife radiosurgery

About 35 percent to 50 percent of patients who undergo brain surgery for OCD will show improvement. Because the surgery is highly specialized, involves the destruction of brain tissue, and is usually considered experimental, it is rarely used. However, for those patients who are severely affected by OCD and for whom no other treatment has worked these are legitimate options.[16]

Most research on OCD has focused on adults, but a few studies have evaluated treatment methods on children and adolescents. One study was a randomized control trials study that followed 75 children with OCD for 10 years. Three treatment groups included: additional CBT (for patients already taking medications), CBT alone, and CBT with medications that were begun at the time of the study. Results showed improvement in all groups, with CBT and medications working in both clinical and research settings.[27]

Another study examined the effects of cognitive therapy (CT) and exposure/response prevention (ERP) in group and individual treatment groups over a two-year period and found that all of the different treatment methods were effective, with less than 10 percent of those who completed treatment suffering a relapse and 50 percent of those who completed treatment fully recovering in two years.[28] CT was tolerated well and reported fewer dropouts than ERP, but for long term results ERP remains firmly established as the best treatment for most OCD patients. Some studies have found that children experienced acceptable results within group as well as individual therapy and used both the CT and ERP techniques. The youngsters who were taking medication maintained their treatment gains over the two-year period as long as they stayed on the medication, but studies showed that medication alone did not resist the tendency to relapse as well as psychotherapy.[28]

Finally, Andres et al. looked at changes in cognitive functioning following combined pharmacotherapy and psychotherapy treatment in children with

OCD, and the findings supported the conclusion that cognitive dysfunction appears to normalize in children with OCD after six months of combined treatment.[29] The researchers found cognitive improvements and partial remissions, both stable outcomes. Studies on children with OCD who have received treatment of any type report improved outcomes and positive results, although findings suggest that it is more challenging to treat OCD in children than in young adults.

POSTTRAUMATIC STRESS DISORDER

The most common treatment of Posttraumatic Stress Disorder (PTSD) is pharmacotherapy; however, the vast majority of sufferers never receive adequate care for this very treatable condition. As in other anxiety-based conditions, adequate care typically involves both medication and psychosocial types of treatment. Past research that has focused on how to prevent people from developing PTSD following a traumatic event has met with dismal results. Neither general counseling nor the use of propanolol (a beta blocker) for 10 days following a trauma prevented the development of PTSD, although the beta blocker did eliminate the physiologic responses to script-driven reminders of trauma.[30] Regarding medical traumas, the use of benzodiazepine tranquilizers following surgery did not help to prevent PTSD, and studies from pediatric burn units have demonstrated that imipramine (a TCA) and fluoxetine (an SSRI) were effective in controlling pain and reducing symptoms of Acute Stress Disorder but ineffective in reducing the probability of developing PTSD.[30]

Although no reliable strategies for preventing PTSD have been identified, several drugs or combinations of medication appear effective in relieving symptoms and in treating people who develop PTSD. The general goals of pharmacotherapy for PTSD are to:

- Reduce or ameliorate target symptoms
- Improve mood and emotional numbing
- Reduce phasic and tonic hyperarousal
- Improve sleep
- Reduce impulsivity
- Reduce psychotic and/or dissociative symptoms
- Treat comorbid Psychiatric Disorders

In general, victims of military trauma were less responsive to most interventions, including medication, than victims of other forms of trauma. Some studies found that trazadone is helpful for sleep but is too sedating to use solely as an antidepressant in treating PTSD. First-line medication treatments for

PTSD often involve benzodiazepine tranquilizers, SSRI and SNRI antidepressants, or other medications used to lessen the arousal and anxiety of PTSD patients or to help deal with the mood symptoms frequently experienced. Patients who have not been responsive to first line pharmacotherapy and are given an adjuvant agent, such as bupropion, will often respond positively, a strong argument for not giving up too quickly when the first treatment is not immediately effective. Studies also found that venlafaxine (an SNRI) was not as effective as sertraline (an SSRI) and that buspirone (an antianxiety medication) looks promising, although supporting research is scant at this time. The benzodiazepines, especially alprazolam, seem helpful with anxiety, but again there is little supportive research.[30]

Agitation and confusion sometimes accompany PTSD, as well as occasional psychotic symptoms, and the use of atypical antipsychotic medications has yielded encouraging results. For example, olanzapine has been effective with PTSD even in the absence of psychotic symptoms, and risperidone showed similar results, including the improvement of comorbid Psychosis. Quetiapine has been effective for Insomnia, but there is no real evidence of any other therapeutic benefits. Finally, mood stabilizers such as lithium, depakote, topamax, and lamictal (the latter two also being anticonvulsant medications) have been used to treat affective lability (extreme mood variability) and to reduce the impulsive and aggressive behaviors sometimes exhibited by PTSD sufferers.[30]

In summary, research and clinical data support a stage-based use of pharmacotherapy in the treatment of Posttraumatic Stress Syndrome:

- First hours: reduce terror and neuronal imprinting with adrenergic blockers.
- First days: reduce sensitization and memory consolidation with adrenergic blockers and/or mood stabilizers.
- First months: reduce symptoms with SSRIs and low-dose trazadone for sleep.
- After the first year: reduce symptoms and comorbidity with SSRIs, adrenergic blockers, and/or mood stabilizers.

Most publicity and advertising about the treatment of PTSD focus primarily on pharmacotherapy. Mansell and Read examined the top 54 websites on PTSD and found that 42 percent of them receive funding from a drug company.[31] It is not surprising, therefore, that much more emphasis was placed on the use of medications to treat PTSD than nonpharmacologic treatment methods. Research studies concluded that the major influence of the drug companies in the mental health field is designed to increase their product sales using a biased presentation of facts rather than to improve general knowledge and treatment, an influence that now also pervades the Internet.[31]

In addition to medication, psychotherapeutic interventions are just as important in the treatment of PTSD. As with most other Anxiety Disorders, the current research is more supportive of CBT than of supportive therapy for PTSD patients, and few systematic studies are looking at other forms of psychosocial treatment.[1] Some providers tried to apply the principles of positive psychology to the treatment of trauma-based disorders, and, while this looks promising, minimal evidence of success exists. Certainly, there is a role for medication in the treatment of PTSD, but we cannot neglect the psychosocial methods in the treatment of PTSD and related disorders.

OTHER CONSIDERATIONS IN TREATING ANXIETY DISORDERS

One of the main areas of concern for providers who are treating patients with Anxiety Disorders is recognizing and treating comorbid conditions, since most people with anxiety problems suffer from more than one psychiatric condition. Most of the research on comorbidity focuses on Mood Disorders, Substance Use Disorders, and other Axis I conditions (Clinical Disorders, see chapter 1). However, we are beginning to recognize the importance of diagnosing and treating Axis II disorders (Personality Disorders). It has been demonstrated that early recognition and treatment of Personality Disorders is very important to predicting treatment outcomes for both Anxiety and Mood Disorders.[32]

In addition to considering comorbid conditions, more recent treatment initiatives are being directed to special groups, including children and the elderly. The use of CBT in reducing anxiety in children is well established, as is the reduction of negative automatic thoughts and better control of anxiety symptoms in youths.[33] Another fascinating study done in the United States and Sweden examined the treatment of Specific Phobia in youths and used three groups: Group I, One-Session Exposure Treatment; Group II, Education/Supportive Treatment; and Group III, Waitlist Control. Results indicated that both treatment groups (Groups I and II) did better than the Waitlist Control, and the One-Session Exposure Treatment was more effective than Education/Support on most measures.[34] Given the pervasiveness and potentially serious implications of childhood Anxiety Disorders, finding new and effective treatments is very important. Authors also found participant modeling, in vivo exposure, and reinforced practice to be helpful when treating anxiety in youths.

Another inventive study reported that therapeutic alliance with parents of youths being treated for Anxiety Disorders was very encouraging, especially since most youths enter into treatment not because they have chosen to but because their parents have decided that it is important. By including the parents in the alliance along with the youngster and the therapist, it was found that the strength of the alliance grew over several sessions. Since it has been established that CBT, along with exposure tasks, is effective in treating Anxiety Disorders in children and adolescents, it is also accepted that, by including parents in sessions, therapeutic alliance treatment is even more effective.[35] This strategy is supported and followed by many therapists, myself included.

Another approach that places parents in the roles of potentially supportive therapeutic allies was conducted by Ginsburg, who developed a prevention type of program for children at high risk for developing Anxiety Disorders.[36] The children were deemed high risk because they came from families in which one or both parents suffered from an Anxiety Disorder. The children and their parents were provided an educational and supportive program designed to help prevent the onset of Anxiety Disorders in children. The treatment group was compared with a waitlist control group, and results demonstrated that, at the point of a one-year follow-up, 30 percent of the children in the control group had developed an Anxiety Disorder, but none of the children in the education/support group had. Of course, no one can say that this type of program will eliminate all future Anxiety Disorders, but there is certainly reason to believe that these types of family-based interventions can be very effective.

Mexican American youth have demonstrated a growing need for treatment of Anxiety Disorders and are one of the most undertreated groups. Even when Mexican American youths agree to treatment, they frequently drop out because the treatment provider does not know how to relate to or treat them. A very thorough study conducted by Wood et al. examined some of the issues in depth and offered suggestions to the schools and school psychologists who deal mostly with these students.[37] First, they note that Mexican American students are the fastest growing group in U.S. schools, and in California more than one-third of public school students are Mexican American. In fact, Mexican Americans are the fastest growing Latino/a group in the United States. Second, they also find that Mexican American families underutilize mental health services and are more likely to drop out of treatment early. Another challenge to providing appropriate mental health treatment is language; about 25 percent of students in California schools are English learners, with 75 percent of those Spanish speaking. Third, Mexican American students are more likely than European American students to face inequities such as poverty and poor health insurance coverage. Clearly, there is a high and largely unfulfilled need for mental health services among Mexican American youths.

The research evidence suggests that CBT is an effective treatment for Mexican American youth suffering from Anxiety Disorders, but there are several principles that can help adapt CBT effectively to these youngsters:

- Principle 1: Learn each family's cultural practices, acculturative status, migration history, language proficiencies and preferences, and other relevant background.
- Principle 2: Collaborate with school staff to alleviate parental apprehension.
- Principle 3: Provide an orientation early to increase family understanding and participation.
- Principle 4: Respect the family's conceptualization and treatment of mental illness to increase acceptance of CBT techniques.
- Principle 5: Establish CBT goals that are valued by the family to improve the working relationship.
- Principle 6: Learn about the cultural context of parenting to facilitate engagement in CBT.
- Principle 7: Engage the extended family in the child's CBT treatment.
- Principle 8: Align CBT techniques with family cultural beliefs and traditions to enhance commitment to treatment.
- Principle 9: Consider whether culturally based conversational norms are masking poor adherence to treatment.
- Principle 10: Remain attuned to the role of acculturation gaps in children's adjustment problems, but consult with cultural experts before addressing this topic with families.

Evidence-based CBT programs for Mexican American students, as well as other diverse clients, may be enhanced by making culturally appropriate adaptations to treatment[37] and delivering quality care to those who need it—a goal we should all embrace.

The elderly is another group that tends to be untreated or inadequately treated for Anxiety Disorders. They appear to respond to medications (especially SSRIs), although some medications may be dangerous (e.g., benzodiazepines, TCAs); the elderly also respond well to CBT. One study offers evidence on a new medication called pregabalin as a potential treatment for GAD. This drug has been licensed for use in the treatment of GAD in the elderly in Europe but not yet in the United States. Pregabalin seems to produce an earlier therapeutic effect (less than two weeks) than antidepressants and was effective in treating both psychological and somatic symptoms of anxiety.[38] It seems to be a safe and effective treatment for GAD in older adults, but more research is needed.

Because many elderly are reluctant to discuss psychological problems, it can be difficult to recognize and respond to their needs. They will often notice physical symptoms first, believing the symptoms are related to a medical issue, and will only talk to their primary care physician about physical ailments that trouble them. Sometimes, it is only the physical conditions that are treated, and the anxiety condition may be missed or ignored. Suggestions for dealing with anxiety issues in the elderly include:

- Relevant questions to ask the patient:
  - Are you worrying or concerned about anything or anybody?
  - Are you concerned about anything that is going on in your life right now?
  - Do you have a hard time putting worrisome thoughts out of your mind?
  - Are there any changes to your normal daily routine and activities?
  - Are you worrying more than usual (are the worries realistic)?
  - Have you started or stopped a new medication recently?
  - How is your overall mood? (Is it normal for them?)
- Identify the nature of physical symptoms:
  - What were you doing when you noticed the chest pain (or other symptom)?
  - What were you thinking about when your heart started to race?
  - When you can't sleep, what is usually going through your head?[39]

It is important to recognize, diagnose, and treat anxiety conditions, but for those who are chronically underserved, it is essential to improve treatment opportunities and train professionals to be aware of sensitive cultural issues. It is easy to avoid or ignore problems that do not seem to directly affect us, but the resulting community and societal challenges will eventually and ultimately affect us all.

SUMMARY

Although several treatment themes are consistent for Anxiety Disorders, there are some subtle but very real differences in how each condition is treated. Making an assessment and appropriate diagnosis is a complex and multifaceted task that requires experience, training, time, and opportunity. Often, the gate to successful treatment is a collaborative effort between the patient, family and friends, treating professionals, schools, and even the workplace. Today, many organizations and employers provide employee assistance programs that provide counseling and guidance services for some problems and referrals or other assistance for more complex issues. Respecting patient confidentiality is essential and can be maintained while coordinating care and consolidating treatment gains. By working together we can provide more effective and appropriate care to those who need it, while respecting patients' rights, values, and preferences.

9

Living with Anxiety Disorders

Anxiety is the rust of life, destroying its brightness and weakening its power.

—Anonymous

WHO NEEDS TREATMENT?

Everyone feels anxious from time to time, but two diagnostically relevant factors set those who need treatment for an Anxiety Disorder apart from those who do not:

- First, do the symptoms produce significant distress to the patient?
- Second, do the symptoms contribute to dysfunction in one or more of the important areas of a person's life (work, relationships, social activities, school, etc.)?

Suffering from a clinical disorder means that the symptoms are consistent with the diagnostic criteria found in *DSM-IV* and significantly affect daily life, not just cause temporary discomfort or a bad day.

Some people will resist treatment by denying their anxiety difficulties or claiming they can deal with it, which explains why some people try to reduce their anxiety symptoms through the use of drugs and/or alcohol. This solution, of course, only exacerbates the symptoms and will lead to new and more complex problems. Several symptoms of anxiety are physical in nature (e.g., racing heart, rapid and shallow breathing, difficulty swallowing, etc.) and are responsible for leading many patients to initially consult with their primary care physician (PCP) expecting to find a physical illness. When trying to decide whether treatment is needed for an Anxiety Disorder, consider listening to those around you—family members, friends, and coworkers may spot problems before you do. The concerns of others might not indicate that you suffer from an Anxiety Disorder, but they might present you with enough questions and a reason to seek a professional opinion.

WHERE TO SEEK TREATMENT

Most people begin the search for a mental health professional by visiting their PCP, who is familiar with their medical history. Often, the PCP initially will prescribe a medication to calm acute symptoms and may issue a referral to a mental health professional if the symptoms do not respond to medication alone. Members of the clergy are often trained to provide basic counseling and are another source of advice and referrals to mental health professionals when needed. The school nurse, guidance counselor, school psychologist, or school social workers are additional important resources for students and their parents. College students can seek assistance or a referral at either their college's counseling center or their academic or residence advisors.

Many companies offer employee assistance programs where employees can seek confidential, short-term counseling or the names of professionals for additional help. The human resources or personnel department at places of employment can be a source of advice and referrals as well. Most medical insurance companies keep a list of participating professionals, usually listed by zip code, that can be accessed via telephone or websites. A state psychological association can refer inquiries to an appropriate psychologist. One can directly call licensed psychologists, who are typically listed in the yellow pages. Psychiatrists are medical doctors and are found under "Physicians" in the telephone book both alphabetically and by specialty. Most county medical societies can make referrals as well. Many counties, hospitals, and communities have outpatient mental health clinics where people can seek psychological or psychiatric assistance, and often they will accept clients of limited means. Colleagues, friends, and family members may know of a competent professional, but be sure to consult with your PCP first. Victims of a crime can call the state office of victim services or the bureau of crime victims and ask if they are eligible to receive services. Veterans of the military can call the local Veterans Administration and ask about available mental health services.

TYPES OF MENTAL HEALTH PROFESSIONALS

How does one choose the appropriate type of mental health professional from the many different titles, professions, and licenses that one might encounter? As a general rule, it is safer to see a professional who is licensed by one's state or relevant licensing body. Each state sets its own professional standards and usually has its own professional licensing board; one state may require a therapist to hold a license to practice in a certain profession, but some states do not. Insurance companies set their own standards for participating providers, requiring proof of degrees, license, continuing education, and training. One way to better understand the covered services and available providers is to call the insurance company and ask. Can you see a psychologist? Psychiatrist? Social Worker? Counselor? Certified Specialist? Lists of providers on websites or given over the telephone may not be up to date, so it is best to check with the individual provider that you might want to see directly. Counseling and psychotherapy are generally covered under the mental or behavioral health portion of insurance coverage and may be limited to a certain number of sessions annually or weekly and deemed medically necessary. Insurance may not cover a particular or chronic diagnosis and may not cover family, marriage, educational, or court-ordered counseling. Drug and alcohol treatment, inpatient or outpatient, may be covered under a different part of the insurance and might be limited to a certain number of sessions or time period. A psychiatrist's services, including medication checks, are usually covered under the medical portion of the insurance and are not subject to the limitations of other mental health services. Some insurance companies manage their own mental health coverage, and others pay a second company to monitor and manage authorizations, claims, and appeals. Some insurance companies require that a patient obtain authorization prior to seeing a mental health provider and expect clients to be aware of such requirements before being seen. Call the company to check on authorization requirements. Typically, a patient should see only one mental health professional for therapy and one psychiatrist or prescribing professional for medication consults. Seeing multiple therapists is discouraged and is counterproductive and confusing for the patient. Insurance companies will usually cover only one mental health professional at a time; this does not include appointments with medical doctors who are providing prescriptions and are covered under medical coverage rather than mental health coverage. The mental health profession offers a variety of services under the following provider titles:

Psychologist: has a doctoral degree, usually a PhD, PsyD, or EdD, and includes such specialties as clinical, counseling, neuropsychology, industrial/organizational, forensic, school, educational, and many others.

Psychiatrist: has an MD (doctor of medicine) or a DO (doctor of osteopathy) degree and additional training for providing mental health services and is licensed to prescribe medications and conduct other medical treatments.

Nurse practitioner (NP), psychiatric nurse practitioner (PNP), or physician's assistant (PA): usually has a four-year college degree or a nursing degree (or both); has additional training in mental health services; and can write prescriptions and provide other medical services but only under the supervision of (or in collaboration with) a physician.

Social worker: has a master's degree in social work, although some have a bachelor's degree in social work and work under supervision in a limited context. There are many different classifications for social workers, including:

LCSW-R: Licensed clinical social worker-R has a master's degree and has met strict requirements, including six years of experience; is often reimbursable by insurance companies; and can practice independently.

LCSW: Licensed clinical social worker replaced the title of clinical social worker (CSW) after September 2004; has a master's degree but without the "R" designation cannot practice independently and is not directly reimbursed by insurance companies.

CSW: Clinical social worker was a term used prior to September 2004 and has a master's degree.

ACSW: Associate clinical social worker has a master's degree.

MSW: Master's degree in social work is the generic degree held by most social workers.

DSW: Doctor of social work is usually in an academic setting involving teaching and research, although can provide direct services to clients as well.

MSN: Master's of science in nursing has additional training to provide specific services to patients.

APRN: Advanced practice registered nurse is a registered nurse who has additional training but not at the master's level.

Psychotherapist: not a regulated or recognized profession; it is a title used by many degree holders or licensed professionals as well as persons without a degree or any professional training.

Counselor/therapist: a title used by many who provide a variety of counseling services including family, marriage, pastoral, guidance, sex, career, school, college, addiction, alcohol, drug; does not require a specific degree or training, although some states license master's-level providers who offer specific counseling services.

Alcohol/drug counselor: a paraprofessional designation that requires certification, training, and/or accreditation and can vary from state to state; can include a college degree or online courses and minimal training; limited to providing counseling only for substance abuse issues unless they hold licenses or certifications in other areas as well.

Clients who are seeking treatment from a licensed professional can be assured that they are receiving care from a provider who has met the standards for education and training and who will be held accountable for meeting ethical and professional standards of care in the profession. In most states, licensed professionals include psychologists, psychiatrists, and social workers. In other states, subdoctoral mental health specialties are licensed to provide services, such as mental health counselors, family counselors, and others.

A psychologist is a doctoral-level mental health provider with a PhD (doctor of philosophy), a PsyD (doctor of psychology), or an EdD (doctor of education). Licensed psychologists who provide mental health services are usually clinical psychologists or counseling psychologists. The PhD degree means that psychologists, in addition to learning about mental health issues and treatments, are trained in theory and do major research in an original area. The PsyD degree focuses more on clinical practice with some exposure to theory and research, but not as intensely. The EdD degree is primarily in education and sometimes includes a counseling degree from a college of education to provide general counseling as well as school-based interventions. Practitioners with an EdD degree are usually trained in theory and research but typically with an educational emphasis.

In general, a psychologist's education begins with a bachelor's degree in any field, although prerequisite courses relevant to the appropriate field of study must be taken. If a person is accepted into a doctoral training program, the education continues with four to six years of doctoral training in a specific field, and areas such as clinical, counseling, or neuropsychology require a full-time one-year internship in an accredited setting as well as a doctoral dissertation, which is an original piece of major research. Sometimes a student will pursue a master's degree prior to entering a doctoral program, but this is not usually required. In some states, psychologists with additional education and supervised experience and who pass a rigorous examination are permitted to prescribe medications. These are very new programs, and there are not many psychologists who have received this training, although programs continue to grow and the numbers of psychologists who qualify for this level of practice is increasing.

Following the completion of doctoral training, a clinical or counseling psychology student must complete a full-time, one-year internship at an approved facility in order to sharpen their clinical skills. To become licensed in most states, in addition to their education and training, a psychologist must receive two years of supervised experience, and one of these years must be after the completion of the internship. Some psychologists who want to specialize in a given field will receive training for two or more years after the internship as part of a postdoctoral fellowship.

A psychologist is specifically trained to provide psychological methods of therapy that focus on the thoughts, feelings, and behaviors of a patient and is the only mental health specialist who is extensively trained in the administration and the interpretation of psychological tests. Some psychologists specialize in the physical or medical issues of behavioral problems or work with those who suffer from physical/medical problems and have secondary psychological issues.

Additional levels of certification are also available to psychologists, such as the National Register of Health Service Providers in Psychology, a list of psychologists who have met appropriate licensing standards and have demonstrated higher levels of training and experience than required by a license alone. Registered providers are held to the highest ethical and practice standards. Since in most states psychologists are not licensed by specialty, the license that is issued to practice is generic. A psychologist who wishes to attain the highest level of specialty certification can go before the American Board of Professional Psychology (ABPP) to be board certified in the chosen field. The initials ABPP following the PhD at the end of a psychologist's name indicate that she has met the highest standards of education, training, and professional and ethical conduct. In addition, these practitioners must pass demanding examinations and have secured supportive professional references.

A psychiatrist is a medical doctor with an MD or DO degree who has completed four years of medical school and a residency in psychiatry—usually an additional three to four years. Further training allows a doctor to specialize in an area such as child and adolescent psychiatry. The psychiatrist is medically and pharmacologically trained and is allowed to write prescriptions and to provide medical services such as conducting physical examinations, ordering medical tests, prescribing medications, and conducting electroconvulsive therapy. Most psychiatrists receive some training in psychotherapy, although this is not their main focus. Many psychiatrists rely on psychiatric nurse practitioners or psychiatric physician assistants, who are allowed to prescribe medications under the supervision of or in collaboration with a licensed psychiatrist. If it is difficult to secure an appointment with a psychiatrist, it is often possible to see a psychiatric nurse practitioner or physician's assistant within the same practice sooner.

Both psychologists and psychiatrists are doctoral-level providers who have received extensive training in their fields and are capable of providing a broad range of services for patients who have mental health needs. Certainly, if a patient needs medication that cannot be provided or followed by the PCP, a psychiatrist is usually the best resource. If a patient needs nonmedical types of treatment or is not sure whether medication is needed, a psychologist is the provider to call for an initial evaluation. Frequently psychologists, psychiatrists, and PCPs collaborate in the treatment of patients, and most patients appreciate their doctors consulting with each other and feel that they are receiving the most responsive care when that happens.

Social work is another mental health profession that provides services such as counseling and psychotherapy to individuals and families, and a social worker can collaborate with a psychiatrist if a patient needs medication. A social worker has either a four-year undergraduate degree in social work or a graduate degree known as a master of social work (MSW), normally a two-year, full-time program. In some states, social workers can practice independently if they are licensed with a master's degree and have a certain amount of experience. They can practice in a number of different areas, including mental health counseling, marriage and family counseling, and drug and alcohol counseling, but often they work under the auspices of an agency or hospital; they can also be required to work under a doctoral-level provider's supervision unless they are licensed to practice independently. This is similar to the model used for physician's assistants and nurse practitioners, who provide medical services under the supervision of a physician. As mentioned above, it is possible to earn a doctoral degree in social work, but it is usually in the field of academia to teach and do research in a specialty area. Most doctoral-level practitioners are also proficient in counseling fields; while the master's-level providers are specifically trained in a specialty area and do not provide services in other areas.

IS TREATMENT WORKING, AND WHEN IS IT COMPLETED?

The effects of treatment are often subtle, and results are sometimes slow to emerge. Determining whether treatment is working can be difficult, but clearly stating the criteria and goals prior to treatment and then tracking progress can help to outline for the patient some of the gains being made, however small they may seem. During the initial consultation, the provider must complete a full assessment, formulate a diagnostic picture, and begin to develop a treatment plan. The therapist then discusses the findings and treatment options with the client, including medication, psychotherapy, or both. The provider should be prepared to discuss the advantages and disadvantages of various treatment options and encourage input from the patient in order to determine the level of understanding, preferences, and expectations. Goals should be realistic and attainable. Methods of evaluating progress and setting a termination target should be clear. For example, challenging a client's statement of "I want to feel better" by asking for specific examples of changes that they would like to see in their daily life would help to clarify for the provider the patient's understanding and expectations of treatment. Goals such as not having to miss work due to anxiety, keeping anxiety levels low enough to be able to accomplish daily tasks, and being in a more positive mood on most days are specific and yet realistic expectations. Because it is difficult to precisely measure subjective criteria, it is helpful if the client can track his progress in small steps toward attainable goals. Consequently, it is vital that patients attend regularly scheduled appointments and avoid missing appointments, which creates gaps in treatment. To discourage last-minute cancellations by patients and to provide emergency appointments when needed, most offices require 24 hours notice to change or cancel an appointment. Just as importantly, providers should inform clients of future dates when they will be unavailable in the office and who will be on call in their place. Most practices now require that patients pay the required copay or coinsurance fee at the time of each visit rather than billing patients later. Not only does this significantly reduce the cost of running an office, but it is an expression of commitment on the part of the patient to the treatment process. Being responsible and remembering the form of payment is often an indication of a patient's personal investment in the treatment.

It is not uncommon for patients and providers to change goals or expectations during treatment as new situations arise, but it is important that they collaboratively discuss the changes and reestablish the new goals, expectations, and criteria. In fact, it is helpful to occasionally revisit these issues during treatment to ensure that the original plan is still appropriate and make modifications if necessary and agreed upon. Sometimes a client or provider will notice that they are not relating well to each other, or the rapport is uncomfortable, which may be due to a client who prefers a therapist of a different gender, age or generation, nationality or culture, in a different office setting, or with a different style of interacting. Not every therapist will be appropriate for every patient, and it is important that a provider give the patient an opportunity to express feelings or doubts in these situations prior to or during the treatment process and be willing to discuss and deal with these issues. Rarely, but importantly, a provider may decide to refer the client to another professional, and this, too, should be discussed with the client, with the options and the advantages and disadvantages explored before a decision is made.

When it appears to either the patient, the professional, or both that the relevant goals have been attained and treatment is completed, the patient and the provider should discuss the option of termination or of continuing with additional treatment. Sometimes a patient will decide to tackle another issue, or the provider recognizes the need for addressing a related problem, and a discussion is necessary to set new goals, clarify expectations, determine criteria, and begin a new phase of treatment. Occasionally, new treatment issues arise, and a patient would be better served by referral to a different provider.

Once the patient feels that the goals have been achieved, the patient and the provider should discuss how termination will occur and the approximate number of visits it will take. Once termination occurs, the therapeutic relationship is ended, usually with the understanding that, if the patient is in need of further assistance, she can call for an appointment in the future.

What happens if goals are not attained and treatment is not completed due to a decision on the part of the client or the provider? Sometimes clients will suddenly drop out of treatment or discuss with the provider their intention to quit before goals are achieved. The provider can outline the recent progress and accomplishments of the client and offer to continue when the client chooses to do so. The provider can also agree to the termination of treatment, in which case the therapist notifies the client and the PCP (or other referring source) in writing that treatment has been stopped as of a certain date and that the patient is no longer under the care of the therapist. If the patient calls again to request continued treatment, it is up to the provider to decide whether restarting the therapeutic relationship or referring the client elsewhere is in the client's best interest. Some medical insurance companies require notification of treatment terminations.

WHAT PATIENTS CAN DO TO HELP THEMSELVES: STRESS MANAGEMENT

The concept of stress is often misunderstood, which is one of the reasons it can be difficult to control. Stress is not something negative that happens to us; rather, it is a neutral psychological and physical response to an external, or sometimes internal, event, which means that anything that happens to us can produce a stress response. Frequently, stress management is an element of formal treatment, the goal being to help the patient to manage his life in healthier and more productive ways. Sometime this requires maintenance treatment (once or twice a month) for people with chronic conditions or who are in chronically stressful situations. Appointments for stress management maintenance can include:

1. Consolidating and reinforcing positive gains
2. Identifying new activities and opportunities
3. Monitoring symptoms and behavior for relapse and tracking less productive patterns of behavior
4. Continuing stress management practices

Regardless of the psychological or medical problems, stress can always worsen or complicate the issues. Most people feel victimized by stress, as though there is nothing they can do about it. An important element of treatment is learning to recognize what you can and cannot control. The Serenity Prayer, which is attributed to theologian Reinhold Niebuhr and is used by Alcoholics Anonymous and other 12-step programs, says it best:

> God, grant me the serenity
> To accept the things I cannot change,
> The courage the change the things I can,
> And the wisdom to know the difference.

The first rule of stress management is to assess the issues in your life that are causing problems and to focus your time and energy only on those things over which you have some control. Learning new ways to deal with the remaining difficult people and situations in your life, rather than trying to fix and change them all, is a less stressful and more sensible way to manage.

The second rule of stress management is to develop a perspective toward perceived problems. The following popular phrase makes that point:

Don't sweat the small stuff, and almost all of it is small stuff.

I have heard this very wise guidance given many times, and it is certainly worth remembering.

Frequently, patients feel completely overwhelmed and as if their lives are out of control. They begin to feel like a victim who is besieged by powers and forces that they cannot combat. When people begin to feel helpless and hopeless, they may experience psychological symptoms such as anxiety or depression. Learning to manage the stress caused by these feelings and the circumstances that produce them is one of the basic fundamentals of stress management. The first step is to identify the source of stress and determine whether it can be either minimized or eliminated. We cannot always directly impact the source of the stress and, instead, must modify our response to it, thereby minimizing the negative effects upon us.

The second step, when feeling overwhelmed, is to review the list of things that need to be done and take care of one or two small items just to get them off the list. Another tactic that can help is to organize chores by time rather than task. Instead of saying, "I have to clean the house," one could say, "I am going to work on the house for two hours and then take a break and do something different." Achieving small goals helps people to feel in control of their surroundings and to combat feelings of helplessness and hopelessness.

The stimulus that produces feelings of stress or anxiety is called a *stressor*. A stressor that produces a negative response is called *distress*, and a stressor that produces a positive response is called *eustress*—not a word most people will recognize because we usually think of stress as something bad. Any changes in our lives, including the positive ones, produce stress, such as graduating from school, starting a new job, having a baby, buying a house, family gatherings, and so on. The net effect of stress upon a person includes both positive and negative types of stress and is cumulative and persistent. Stress does not simply disappear when a stressful situation is concluded; rather, the effects of stress can persist over time and may affect us physically, psychologically, and emotionally long after the stressful situation has passed.

Managing anxiety and stress involves taking proactive steps before something forces us to slow down or take medical leave due to health changes such as illness, heart attack, stroke, depression, or anxiety. Strategies for effectively managing stress include:

- Exercise
  - Do it regularly (at least three or four times per week).
  - Vary exercise activities; do things that you enjoy.
  - Start slowly and build up.
  - Check with your physician regarding exercise.
  - Schedule exercise times on your calendar before other appointments; do not make excuses—this needs to be a priority.
- Relaxation
  - Learn techniques for deep muscle relaxation, meditation, or yoga; CDs are available that teach relaxation and other related techniques.
  - Practice regularly (three to seven times per week).
  - Learn regulated breathing techniques.
- Time management
  - Use a formal or informal organizing strategy such as a calendar, journal, lists, a cell phone, a personal digital assistant, or a portable computer.
  - Prioritize.
  - Do not overbook yourself—schedule time for rest.
  - Minimize time wasters like TV and video games.
  - Schedule short breaks throughout the day.
  - Organize chores by time rather than task.
- Recreation
  - Do things just for fun.
  - Do not try to convince yourself that chores and work are recreation unless you truly enjoy doing them.
  - Enjoy activities alone (hobbies, reading, listening to or playing music).
  - Enjoy activities with a significant other (take a walk, go on a date, take a day or weekend trip, go on vacation).
  - Enjoy activities with family or friends.

Additional recommendations for dealing with anxiety and stress include:

- Stay socially involved and active—keep in touch with the people who are important to you, but do not overdo it.
- Minimize or eliminate caffeine and other stimulants.
- Minimize or eliminate depressant drugs like alcohol—they may initially have a calming effect, but when they wear off, intensified anxiety or panic attacks will return.

- Regulate sleep patterns
  - Get up at about the same time each day.
  - Do not extend sleep on weekends by more than an hour.
  - Get enough sleep.
    - Do you wake up rested without an alarm clock?
    - Do you feel tired during the day?
    - Most Americans are sleep deprived, and it takes a toll on your health.
  - Do not nap during the day if it interferes with your ability to fall and stay asleep at night—rest periods are fine; if you do need a nap, do so at the same time each day and only for an hour.
- Develop good nutrition
  - Talk to your physician or a nutritionist.
  - Do not overeat carbohydrates as found in white pasta, bread, potatoes, and other starches.
  - Eat lots of vegetables, fruits, and proteins; they are your friends.
  - Good nutrition is not punishment.
    - Eat fresh food rather than canned or processed.
    - Minimize unhealthy snacks.
    - Eat meals and healthy snacks regularly; five or six small meals or snacks each day is healthier than three large meals
    - Control portion sizes, use a smaller plate.
    - Drink lots of water.
    - Minimize saturated and animal fats, fried food, margarine, and butter.

I give my patients the strong message that their treatment and recovery are largely in their hands—I can help, but they have to do the daily work. The more they do, the sooner they will notice improvements and the better they will feel. The older generations had some good advice: "Remember, moderation in all things." Do not overeat, overwork, overspend, overexercise, oversocialize, overdrink, and so on. Recreational activities such as gambling and hobbies should be carefully monitored to avoid developing new problems. Successful management of anxiety and stress requires following a treatment plan and initiating changes. People who suffer from Anxiety Disorders have the ability, with assistance from a trained mental health provider, to establish new patterns to improve their life, to feel better, and to be physically and mentally healthier.

10

Somatoform Disorders

See, I told you I was sick.
— Anonymous, epitaph on the headstone of a confirmed hypochondriac

Somatoform Disorders are a group of conditions characterized by physical symptoms suggestive of a medical illness but in reality represent a Psychiatric Disorder. This is quite different from mental illnesses like Depression, Anxiety, or Psychoses, where physical symptoms are a *result* of the problem. In Somatoform Disorders, the physical symptoms *are* the problem, with a distinct psychological component and no other medical explanation for them. History provides ample evidence of psychological or mental factors influencing physical functions, but it was not until the 20th century that scientifically sound explanations were developed, and we will explore some of them later in this chapter. Most people—especially those with chronic medical conditions—can easily link their recurring physical symptoms with stressful experiences. That is, when under stress, the physical symptoms are either precipitated or worsened. Although the presenting problem may be medical, the surfacing physical symptoms may be entirely or predominantly precipitated by a stressful condition or event. It is not unusual for a psychologist or a psychiatrist to receive a referral from a physician when the physician is unable to establish an adequate medical basis for a patient's physical symptoms and needs an evaluation to determine the possibility of contributing psychological factors. In many somatoform conditions, the pathophysiology is unknown—this means there is no clear understanding of the underlying physiological reasons for the symptoms.[1] These disorders are not rare; more than 12 percent of young adults have reported at least one Somatoform Disorder during their lifetime.[2]

Patients with a primary Somatoform Disorder exhibit a heightened awareness of normal bodily sensations and, if paired with a cognitive predisposition
to interpret these sensations as an illness, can produce conditions that are
similar to an illness but are based on faulty interpretations and/or exaggera-
tions of normal bodily functions. Autonomic nervous system arousal may be
high in some patients and can lead to tachycardia (rapid heartbeat) or gastric
hypermotility (nausea, diarrhea). Heightened arousal also may induce muscle
tension and pain associated with other muscular hyperactivity such as muscle
tension headaches.[1]

In the past, when a person had an unexplained medical problem, it was
called *psychosomatic* and was assumed to be a direct structural or physiological
change in the body derived from psychological factors. Later, the term *somatization* referred to the direct somatic (physical) expression of psychological
distress,[3] but today this term is used much more specifically as a diagnostic
category. To diagnose a Somatoform Disorder, a provider must rule out any
general medical conditions and verify that the physical symptoms are not
signs of a different psychological illness.

MALINGERING AND FACTITIOUS DISORDERS

Ruling out Malingering and Factitious Disorders is one of the challenges
in diagnosing somatoform types of symptoms. Both involve the feigning and
conscious fabrication of physical symptoms for the purpose of avoiding a difficult situation or of benefiting in some way. Malingering is the fabrication of
symptoms to obtain external benefit, although it is sometimes difficult to recognize. For example, children will challenge their parents with stomachaches
that only appear on school mornings or on the day of a big test or school
outing. In cases of malingering, we look for patterns that indicate the recurrence of avoiding difficult situations or benefits to be gained, such as financial
(absent from work with pay, injury lawsuit) or free time to play.

Factitious Disorders differ from Malingering in that the person consciously
pretends to have an illness in order to obtain psychological benefits from
being in the sick role and enjoying others' attention, time, and vigilance. In
1951 the sociologist Talcott Parsons suggested four elements that patients
demonstrate when trying to fulfill the sick role[4]:

1. Unable to will themselves back to good health and must be cared for.
2. View their sickness as something negative and want to get well.
3. Seek medical care and must be compliant with medical treatment.
4. Feel they are exempted from normal responsibilities.

Malingering and Factitious Disorders are neither new nor reserved for
modern times. As far back as the ancient Greeks, records reveal people feign-

ing illness for a variety of reasons,[5] but most of the systematic research dates back to the middle of the 20th century. An article by Asher in the British medical journal *Lancet* introduced a particular type of Factitious Disorder called Munchausen's Syndrome after the Baron von Munchausen, who was a character in German literature famous for exaggerating his exploits.[6] Munchausen's Syndrome is a severe, chronic, Factitious Disorder, but, unlike a pure" Factitious Disorder, it is combined with antisocial behavior. Thus, Munchausen's Syndrome is a specific type of Factitious Disorder but is slightly different from the basic form of the disorder. A variant of this condition is called Munchausen's by proxy, when a parent or guardian feigns or even causes medical problems in their child in order to receive vicarious benefits from the child's condition.

The diagnosis of Factitious Disorder requires the intentional creation of physical and/or psychological signs or symptoms for the main benefit of occupying the sick role and with no other obvious external incentives for being sick. People will employ a number of methods to create the impression that they are sick: giving a false medical history; fabricating clinical and laboratory results; and taking medications or substances that produce symptoms, such as inducing vomiting, creating infections, or preventing wounds from healing.

A type of Factitious Disorder that resembles Munchausen's Syndrome usually involves men patients who display chronic factitious symptoms and associated antisocial traits such as pathological lying. They tend to have few relationships and minimal social supports; will typically wander from hospital to hospital for help; and usually will be familiar with hospital procedures, which they can use to their advantage.[7] The regular type of Factitious Disorder involves mostly women and does not display the pathological lying or wandering from hospital to hospital; these patients usually stay within the same medical community, where they are well known and have a stable support system, employment, a history of working in medically related fields, usually accept mental health treatment, and show improvement from this treatment.[8] Their Factitious Disorder often develops in response to a stressful situation; when the stress is relieved, they often return to normal functioning.[9]

The more common comorbid conditions associated with Factitious Disorder are Borderline and Narcissistic Personality Disorders[10] and Substance Abuse Disorders.[11] Similar to Munchausen's Syndrome, Factitious Disorder can also occur by proxy. This involves the intentional creation or feigning of psychological or physical symptoms in another person under their care. The motivation is to assume the sick role by proxy, with no other external incentives, and the behavior cannot be better explained by any another psychological condition.

The epidemiology of Factitious Disorder is difficult to determine since patients cover up their true problem and will seek help from multiple providers, none of whom have a complete clinical history. The range of reported incidence is 0.3 percent to 9.3 percent, depending upon the setting and the study reviewed. In many situations, people will do something to artificially raise their temperature in order to give the impression of an infection or illness.[2]

Difficulties with diagnosing a Factitious Disorder include eliminating other genuine, rare, or complex medical or psychological issues, Somatoform Disorders, and Substance Abuse issues[12] as well as determining whether a real medical illness was induced and remembering that even people with Factitious Disorder do become legitimately ill like everyone else.

In terms of the etiology of Factitious Disorder, several physical and psychological factors include genetics, the environment, or a combination of both. In some cases a childhood developmental disturbance can be related to the onset of Factitious Disorder. Children who suffer from serious illnesses or who have a family member who is seriously ill may be at higher risk for this condition. Other possible factors include past anger with the medical profession, a past significant relationship with a health care provider, and the existence of a Factitious Disorder in a parent.[12] Some patients may create an illness or condition to compensate for an underlying deficit or insecurity and often assume a psychodynamic basis for the condition, which means a possible unconscious determinant of the Factitious Disorder.

The goal of treating Factitious Disorder involves minimizing the potential damage to the patient and the health care system as well as helping the individual to recover from the condition. Strategies include:

1. Identifying and treating comorbid medical conditions.
2. Avoiding unnecessary procedures.
3. Encouraging patients to seek mental health treatment.
4. Providing support for the treating health care professionals.[2]

Following the publication of Asher's[6] article, it was typical for clinicians to confront their patients with their suspicion of Factitious Disorder, and the patient would usually refuse to return and would find a different provider.[13] Eisendrath suggests an approach that respects a patient's confidentiality and sensitivity to this information:

1. Inexact interpretation—the clinician interprets the underlying psychodynamics without presenting the diagnosis of Factitious Disorder to the patient.
2. Therapeutic double-bind—the clinician presents a new medical intervention for the patient's illness and offers the possibility of a Factitious Disorder but stresses that if it is a genuine medical problem, the treatment will work effectively.[13]

Treatment of a person with Factitious Disorder is never simple, since the involvement of multiple providers challenges the effective coordination of treatment. Medications alone do not seem to be helpful, although they may be significant in treating comorbid disorders or symptoms that are not related to the Factitious Disorder. Research suggests that long-term psychotherapy produces positive results; however, most patients with Factitious Disorder resist mental health treatment.[2]

HYPOCHONDRIASIS

Hypochondriasis is a condition that is often misunderstood or is a topic for humor. Although we all are concerned to some extent about our health and worry occasionally about an illness, the level of concern experienced by a hypochondriac is an intense preoccupation with the fear of contracting or suffering from a serious disease based upon the misinterpretation of normal bodily sensations. To diagnose someone with this condition, the patient has to have had the symptoms of the disorder for at least six months. Hypochondriacs do not have a simple headache—they assume it is a stroke or a brain tumor. They do not have indigestion—they assume it is stomach cancer or another serious disease. Despite appropriate medical evaluations and reassurance, the hypochondriac experiences persistent and clinically significant distress or impairment in social, occupational, or other important areas of functioning. Some patients possess the ability to view their own concerns as excessive and irrational, and others are incapable of having true insight into their condition.

Children are rarely diagnosed with Hypochondriasis, but it can emerge during adolescence or young adulthood. One study found that, in a psychiatric outpatient clinic, 69.2 percent of children reported somatic symptoms. Is this indicative of a possible basis for developing Hypochondriasis later? Or are children unable to identify and label symptoms that are not considered physical, such as depression, lack of emotion or focus, and mood swings? In adults, the prevalence depends on the population studied and the type of diagnostic interview techniques that are used. In one sample drawn from 15 mental health centers around the world, it was found that 0.8 percent of patients were diagnosed with Hypochondriasis, but in the primary care setting about 3 percent were described as having this condition.[2] This may be due to the fact that most Hypochondriacs see their problems as medical and are more likely to be seen in the primary care setting than in a mental health practice.

Hypochondriasis tends to run in families and was found in 7.7 percent of first-degree relatives with this condition. These relatives reported a high rate of comorbid Anxiety, Depressive Disorders, and other Somatoform Disorders, as well as a substantial rate of physical and psychological impairment. Further, they took advantage of health services more often than the average person but were less satisfied with the services.[2]

A person with Hypochondriasis experiences an abnormal preoccupation with health issues and avoiding germs, and they have an unusual and largely exaggerated concern for contracting diseases. They studiously monitor bodily processes and misinterpret or overinterpret benign symptoms to indicate the presence of a severe condition. Regardless of assurances by health professionals and others, they continue to believe that people are not telling them the truth or their grave illness has yet to be discovered and diagnosed. These patients seem to believe that "health" means being totally symptom free and often shop around for a doctor who will agree with them or "correctly" diagnose and fix them, which is a rare occurrence. Interestingly, these patients do not usually demonstrate excessive anxiety, nor do they seem to be in poor health as judged by medical professionals. Usually, Hypochondriasis is associated with deteriorating interpersonal relationships since the patient's symptoms will almost always be more important than their other responsibilities. From their point of view, "It's not my fault—I'm sick."

Hypochondriasis can exist on its own or as a primary condition or as a disorder secondary to another psychiatric disorder (Depression, Generalized Anxiety Disorder, Obsessive-Compulsive Disorder). It is vital to rule out or diagnose insidious and long-term, slow-onset conditions (e.g., multiple sclerosis), which may present as a Somatoform Disorder prior to any medical signs emerging. It is also important to rule out other Psychiatric Disorders, including:

1. Somatoform Disorders
2. Affective Disorders with somatic symptoms (Depression)
3. Anxiety Disorders (usually have physical symptoms)
4. Psychoses
5. Obsessive-Compulsive Disorder (often comorbid with Hypochondriasis)
6. Malingering and Factitious Disorder

Lower socioeconomic status, family conflicts, health issues, and obesity are factors often associated with multiple somatic symptoms, as well as having a genetic disposition to developing a Somatoform Disorder. Data suggest that higher levels of family stress and parental somatic symptoms predict higher levels of somatic symptoms in children. Cognitive abilities and impaired verbal communication also can be contributing factors. For example, an underlying unconscious conflict, wish, or need may seek expression and be converted to a physical symptom without the person being aware of the actual basis for the symptom. The psychodynamic theorists assume that the repression of the unwanted memory maintains anxiety at a low level and continues the probability of the patient expressing only the physical symptoms rather than dealing with the repressed issues or the anxiety. Evidence suggests that victims of childhood physical and/or sexual abuse are more likely to develop Somatoform and Dissociative Disorders.[2]

The learning theorists look to reinforcement patterns and modeling to explain the origin of conditions like Hypochondriasis. If a child is rewarded for sick behavior by gaining more attention, staying at home with a parent, and avoiding unpleasant situations like school, then they are, in fact, being rewarded for fulfilling the sick role. Most parents are aware of this ploy and struggle to give their attention only to legitimate symptoms. If children observe others being sick and gaining attention, then they learn to mimic being sick in order to experience similar advantages and are not aware of what they are doing; since it is practiced and reinforced, it then becomes a part of feeling normal for them.[2]

Research has shown that some children have difficulty expressing their emotions and rely primarily upon physical symptoms to display their distress. High-achieving children who try to meet parental expectations may be unable to tell their parents that they are under too much pressure and may pretend to get sick as a consequence. In some families, expressing emotions is not encouraged, but being sick is tolerated. Thus, children may unconsciously learn to express distress in only physical ways. Family systems theorists feel that somatization patterns such as Hypochondriasis may originate from specific family patterns and processes, and that the child's physical symptoms are actually functional in the maintaining of homeostasis within the family.[2]

Certain environmental and cultural factors have been linked to the development of Hypochondriasis, especially when adequate care is not provided and the culture does not encourage the expression of emotional symptoms. Emerging research links childhood adversity to the development of adult Hypochondriasis. One study of adults found that patients with Hypochondriasis reported having experienced many more traumatic events during their childhood and more substance abuse than did the patients in the control group. Also, parental overconcern about a child's health was positively correlated with a child developing Hypochondriasis later as an adult.[2]

Treating Hypochondriasis is difficult and complex due to the need to treat legitimate medical illnesses and to the fact that patients will blame physicians for not being competent enough to discover the real cause of their symptoms. The goal of treatment is for patients to learn to better control their fear of serious illnesses and their symptoms. Educating patients about Hypochondriasis, as well as other conditions they fear may have developed, is important in allaying suspicions that the providers believe they are making it up or that it is all in their head. Having a comfortable, trusting, and supportive relationship with a health (and mental health) provider is the basis for effective treatment. In addition to psychodynamic therapy aiding patients in the discovery of underlying conflicts and factors, several other approaches such as cognitive-behavioral therapy are well supported in the literature. The more structured behavioral approaches and family therapy help to address family communication patterns and conflicts that might underlie a condition, and patients can learn to cope with stress more effectively through relaxation techniques, cognitive restructuring, and refocusing techniques.[2]

Medication is often effective in treating Hypochondriasis, and antidepressants are used in about 40 percent of cases. Selective serotonin reuptake inhibitors are most frequently prescribed and are most likely to help with comorbid conditions such as Depression or Anxiety Disorders.[2] One of the major problems involved with the use of medication is that patients with Hypochondriasis will read about every possible side effect on the list from the pharmacy and think they are experiencing all or most of them. Typically, patients with Hypochondriasis are only seeking a medical explanation for their symptoms and are reluctant to take medication unless it will clearly and unambiguously lead to a cure.

SOMATIZATION DISORDER

In the past, the diagnosis of Somatization Disorder required only the presentation of physical symptoms that have no apparent physical cause. Today, we use specific criteria including a *chronic, severe* disorder that is characterized by many different and recurring physical symptoms that cannot be fully explained by a physical disorder. Somatization Disorder does not involve imaginary symptoms but rather real symptoms that result from a physical problem, including pain, digestive problems, sexual or urinary difficulties, and neurological factors, as well as psychological factors. The patient usually complains of a wide variety of symptoms, such as headache, nausea, diarrhea, constipation, and fatigue, which have been experienced over several years or longer.

Historically, there is evidence of Somatization Disorder as far back as pre-Hippocratic Egypt, and it was attributed to the uterus becoming dislodged and traveling through the body, where it would cause symptoms. This disorder was mostly identified in women during their childbearing years, a theory that persisted for many centuries. Breuer and Freud (and others) called this disorder *hysteria*" (note the root of the word hysteria and the term *hysterectomy*) and assumed that psychodynamic factors were responsible for producing the physical symptoms.[14] In the more recent past, the term *conversion* was reserved for pseudo-neurological complaints, and the term *somatization* was used for bodily symptoms and considered an expression of neurosis. This condition has also been referred to as Briquet's Syndrome. According to the *DSM-IV-TR*,[15] the specific diagnostic criteria for Somatization Disorder include:

1. A history of physical complaints, beginning before the age of 30 and occurring over a period of years, that results in the significant impairment in various important areas of functioning or in seeking treatment.

2. Each of the following criteria must be met with individual symptoms occurring at any time during the disturbance:
   a. Four pain symptoms
   b. Two gastrointestinal symptoms
   c. One sexual symptom
   d. One pseudo-neurological symptom
3. The person must also present with one of the following:
   a. After appropriate investigation, the above symptoms cannot be fully explained by a known medical condition or be the direct effects of a substance.
   b. When there is a related general medical condition, the physical complaints or resulting social or occupational impairment are in excess of what would be expected from the medical findings.
4. The symptoms are not intentionally feigned or produced, as in Malingering or Factitious Disorder.

Patients with this condition frequently suffer from Mood Disorders, Anxiety Disorders, and Personality Disorders and are often excessively dependent upon others. Although patients do not intentionally produce symptoms, they sometimes enjoy the comfort and attention that then helps them to avoid situations that they would rather escape. However, the symptoms can also prevent the patient from participating in and enjoying the activities that are important to them.[16]

Somatization Disorder tends to run in families and is predominantly found in women. Symptoms usually emerge during adolescence or young adulthood and are often described as "unbearable," "beyond description," or "the worst imaginable" and can vary widely or involve any part of the body. Distinct symptom patterns occur within different cultures, which lend credence to the idea that a psychological component is involved with this disorder in addition to medical issues. Patients often demand help and emotional support and become angry when they feel that no one is meeting their needs. Often dissatisfied with their medical care, they go from doctor to doctor seeking medical tests and treatments and are usually resistant to any psychological interpretations of their symptoms or mental health treatment. This disorder is different from other somatoform conditions due to the variety of symptoms, the involvement of multiple organ systems, and its persistence over many years.[16]

Treatment for Somatization Disorder is never simple or easy, since medical treatments alone will not adequately address all of the symptoms. However, psychotropic medications can help in treating comorbid conditions such as Depression or Anxiety. Research suggests that cognitive-behavioral therapy and other behavioral treatments may help, but the primary challenge is convincing patients to remain in and comply with treatment. It is most important, therefore, that clients develop a trusting relationship with their mental health professional and with their physician.[16] Prognostically, Somatization

Disorders do not respond well to treatment and fluctuate and persist over a person's lifetime. Treatments rarely relieve symptoms completely for a significant length of time, and patients sometimes become depressed and suicidal.[16]

CONVERSION DISORDER

Most of the research in the late 19th and early 20th centuries on Conversion Disorder was conducted by Charcot and his colleagues in France, along with Breuer and Freud in Austria. Freud became interested in "hysteria" as a consulting neurologist working with Josef Breuer, his mentor; Freud continued his studies in France with Charcot and others. During this period, the term *hysteria* indicated that there were underlying, although unclear, emotional factors that led to the physical symptoms. As Freud developed a complex theory and treatment method for dealing with this unusual and difficult condition, more research and professional literature addressed the issues surrounding it.

A person with Conversion Disorder experiences symptoms or deficits in the areas of voluntary, motor, or sensory functioning that are suggestive of, and yet not fully explained by, a neurological or other general medical condition and are not the direct result of substance use. The specific diagnostic criteria include:

1. One or more symptoms or deficits affecting voluntary motor or sensory functioning that suggest a neurological or general medical condition
2. Psychological factors associated with the physical symptoms that are preceded by conflict or stressors
3. Symptoms not intentionally produced or feigned
4. Symptoms not explained by
   a. General medical condition
   b. Direct effects of substances
   c. Culturally sanctioned behavior or experience
5. Symptoms that cause distress, impair functioning, or require medical evaluation
6. Symptoms not limited to pain or sexual dysfunction, not part of a Somatization Disorder, and not part of another mental condition
7. Must specify if:
   a. Motor symptoms or deficits
   b. Sensory symptoms or deficits
   c. Seizures or convulsions
   d. With mixed presentation[15]

Additional research proposes the idea of conversion hallucinations, where a person has perceptual experiences of symptoms that are not detectible by others. However, these hallucinatory experiences are not part of a psychotic process, and there are no other psychotic symptoms. The hallucinations observed in patients with this condition are typically naïve, childish, and fantastic.[2]

For many years Conversion Disorder was considered a rare disorder and a product of the repressive Victorian era in Europe. It was also viewed as an outgrowth of the new psychoanalytic therapies, which tended to attract this type of patient and to encourage therapists to liberally apply this diagnosis. However, findings today suggest that the condition is not as rare as once thought and that it is frequently misdiagnosed or missed altogether. Depending upon the study reviewed, some estimate that Conversion Disorder accounts for 5 percent to 14 percent of all hospital admissions and in the range of 5 percent to 24 percent for psychiatric outpatient appointments. Another estimation suggests that patients with Conversion Disorder are responsible for 1 percent to 3 percent of psychiatric referrals, 4 percent of neurological outpatient referrals, and 1 percent of neurological admissions.[2]

The onset of Conversion Disorder usually occurs from late childhood (not before the age of 10) to early adulthood,[17] although occasionally it can emerge past the age of 35 or, in a few rare cases, in the ninth decade of life.[18] Individual conversion symptoms are generally self-limiting and do not lead to physical changes or disabilities such as muscle atrophy or permanent sensory or muscular changes. Marital, relationship, and occupational difficulties are not as common among those with Conversion Disorder compared to those with Somatization Disorder.[19]

Determining the differential diagnosis of Conversion Disorder can be complex, since true medical issues must first be evaluated and either fully treated or eliminated. For example, vague neurological symptoms may be similar to those in Conversion Disorder but could represent a serious medical issue. Although symptoms are not consciously presented, there is always the possibility that a Malingering or Factitious Disorder exists. Historically, one of the defining characteristics in some, but not all, patients with Conversion Disorder is *la belle indifference*, which means they have a "beautiful indifference" to their symptoms.[20] However, it is also true that other patients will show the same indifference to an actual serious medical condition.[21]

Causes for Conversion Disorder remain elusive, since the origin of a patient's symptoms is difficult to establish. It is assumed that psychological conflicts or problems are the basis of this disorder and are converted into physical symptoms. Also, the physical symptoms seem to reduce feelings of anxiety, but this is difficult to support since many people with Conversion Disorder are highly anxious. Many clinicians will try to determine the symbolic basis of the physical symptoms in order to determine the underlying meaning and unconscious origin of the symptoms, but this process is highly inferential and could lead to unreliable judgments.[22] Further, the psychological overinterpretation of symptoms that represent occult (hidden) medical conditions could lead to misdiagnosis and the neglect or delay of appropriate treatment.[2]

A preexisting Personality Disorder (e.g., Histrionic Personality Disorder) may predispose a patient to develop conversion symptoms.[2] Others with

Conversion Disorder have disturbed sexuality,[23] and one-third of patients report a history of sexual abuse—especially incest.[2] Psychosocial factors are assumed to play a role in the development of this disorder, although sometimes indirectly, and many patients have chaotic domestic or occupational situations. Many reside in rural areas and are medically unsophisticated, and some will model their symptoms after patients with real neurological problems.[2] Some researchers propose a genetic connection, since conversion symptoms are frequently found in the relatives of people with Conversion Disorder,[24] although this, too, may be based on modeling and the reinforcement of symptomatic behavior. Another consideration is that a patient's presentation of symptoms is not usually an accurate portrayal of the true symptoms but rather what he thinks the symptoms should be like. Thus, the symptoms are similar but subtly different from the established neurologic symptoms.

Symptoms frequently found in Conversion Disorder include:

- Paralysis of the arm or leg
- Loss of sensation in a part of the body
- Seizures
- Loss of special senses such as hearing or sight

It is common for symptoms to emerge following a distressing or a traumatic social or psychological event, usually a once-in-a-lifetime occurrence, although the condition itself can be chronic or sporadic. Typically, episodes are brief, and symptoms abate within two weeks if a person is hospitalized. In 20 percent to 25 percent of patients, symptoms will recur within one year; in some patients, symptoms may be chronic.[16]

It is difficult to evaluate the effectiveness of treatment in patients with Conversion Disorder, because symptoms usually diminish on their own within a few weeks regardless of the type of treatment. When mental health providers first began to formally treat Conversion Disorder, the symptoms were eliminated by the use of suggestion or hypnosis but also were treated with free association or other psychoanalytic procedures.[2] It was challenging to determine whether the therapeutic response was due to spontaneous remission, placebo effect, or to something else. Presently, some providers recommend long-term, insight-oriented psychodynamic therapy,[25] but most advocate a more pragmatic and shorter-term approach, especially for acute cases.[2] In most acute cases, the removal of the symptoms is the main goal, and the amount of distress or disability the patient is suffering will provide the incentive for treatment.[25] If there is minimal distress or pressure, more conservative approaches such as reassurance, support, and suggestion are usually most effective.[25] Although true chronicity or disability is rare, it is important for symptoms to be resolved quickly to avoid the risk of recurrence or chronic disability.[26]

If symptoms do not respond to conservative therapy, other approaches such as narcoanalysis (using amobarbital or another drug), hypnosis, or behavior therapy can be used. Narcoanalysis refers to the use of a narcotic drug, or something similar, to induce a state of hyper-relaxed suggestibility, where people are more compliant with suggestion. This is similar to hypnosis but involves the use of drugs to make people more pliant and suggestible. Although their effects are unpredictable and are unreliable, these types of drugs are commonly (mostly in movies, on television, or in the media) known as "truth serum" or "truth drugs." Occasionally, some more extreme forms of therapy will show positive results with Conversion Disorder (e.g., antipsychotic medications, lithium, electroconvulsive therapy), but there is not much supportive research, and most of the reports are anecdotal. In addition, conversion symptoms may be inadvertently resolved during the treatment of a comorbid mental disorder such as Schizophrenia or Bipolar Disorder.[2] In chronic cases, long-term psychotherapy may be warranted and could involve psychodynamic or other types of therapy.

PAIN DISORDER

Patients with Pain Disorders suffer chronic, severe, and often uncontrollable pain that is affected by subjective physical and psychological factors. Although pain is typically a warning sign of real or impending tissue damage, it can sometimes be exacerbated by psychological issues. A minor pain that is based on a clear physical cause and can be treated with medication or other therapies is not a complicated issue. However, determining the course of treatment when pain is the result of both physical and psychological factors is more challenging.

Diagnostically, a Pain Disorder is determined when physical pain is the patient's predominant complaint; is not intentionally produced (as in Malingering or Factitious Disorder); and there is the assumption that psychological factors have a significant role in the onset, severity, exacerbation, or maintenance of the pain. According to the *DSM-IV-TR*,[15] the diagnostic criteria for Pain Disorder are:

1. Pain in one or more anatomical sites, is the predominant focus of the patient complaints, and is sufficiently severe enough to warrant clinical attention.
2. The pain causes significant distress or impairment in social, occupational, or other important areas of functioning.
3. Psychological factors appear to have a significant role in the Pain Disorder.
4. Symptoms are not intentionally produced.
5. The pain is not due to or better explained by another psychological condition and does not meet the diagnostic criteria for Dyspareunia.

6. The diagnosis should specify whether the pain is primarily due to psychological factors or to general medical *and* psychological factors.
7. The diagnosis should specify whether the condition is acute (less than six months) or chronic (more than six months).

Pain is a common patient complaint and is the predominant symptom in more than half of all general hospital admissions. In the United States, 10 percent to 15 percent of adults are on work disability due to back pain, and pain is present in as many as 38 percent of psychiatric inpatient admissions and 18 percent of psychiatric outpatient admissions. Patients who are diagnosed with Pain Disorder are quite diverse, and there is a noticeable variability in the course of each condition. It was found that, in patients who have suffered from their pain condition for less than six months, the prognosis is very good for a full remission. However, in those whose pain is more chronic, the prognosis is not as encouraging.[2]

In terms of comorbidity, it is not surprising that Depression often accompanies chronic pain conditions, especially in patients with facial pain, and antidepressant medications often ease the pain, regardless of whether the patient is depressed. Other psychiatric conditions, external stress and conflict, as well as any reinforcement received (avoiding work, gaining sympathy, support, etc.) can also influence Pain Disorder. One study found that a good predictor of therapeutic improvement is whether a patient is employed at the outset of treatment.[27] It has also been demonstrated that chronicity is more likely to be present in patients with certain personality traits such as passivity and dependence.[2]

When treating Pain Disorder, the clinician must avoid saying or doing anything to perpetuate and promote pain-related behavior.[28] Most pain specialists today recommend taking medications on a fixed interval schedule and avoiding sedative-antianxiety medications and opioids.[2] However, if comorbid Depression exists, it must be treated with antidepressant medication. Patients should seek professionals who are experienced in dealing with pain conditions and are familiar with the various treatment approaches, especially with chronic pain patients, where a multidisciplinary team approach (specialists from different professions) is the most effective treatment model. Some tips for treating pain include:

1. Pharmacotherapy is the primary approach in reducing *acute* pain.[29]
2. Maintaining functioning is the primary goal in chronic pain conditions, since reducing the pain may not be possible.
3. Relaxation and stress management, behavioral therapies, and cognitive-behavioral therapy (or other nonpharmacological psychological therapies) are helpful, particularly for chronic pain patients.
4. Pharmacotherapy for chronic conditions includes the following guidelines:

a. Avoid opioids, if possible.
b. Antidepressant medications sometimes relieve (and may eliminate) pain even in patients without Depression. Duloxetine, an antidepressant, is effective in relieving peripheral neuropathic pain, particularly in diabetic patients. Amitriptyline, another antidepressant, is effective at low doses for some Pain Disorders.
c. Nonsteroidal analgesic medications, including aspirin or acetaminophen.
d. Anticonvulsants, like carbamazepine.
e. Antidepressant medications for neuropathic pain, headache, facial pain, fibrocitis, and arthritis (osteoarthritis and rheumatoid arthritis as well).
f. Opioids are rarely used, and the goal is a measurable outcome such as increased function rather than pain control. Use milder opioids as the first line and then move to stronger ones, if needed.
g. Acupuncture, transcutaneous electrical nerve stimulation, and massage may help some patients and are low risk.
h. Trigger point injections, nerve blocks, and surgical ablation, if consistent with the underlying medical condition, may also be warranted and helpful in some patients.

Pain Disorder is a persistent and expensive condition, often requiring extensive diagnostic procedures and lengthy, perhaps constant, treatment. Chronic low back pain is a common and frequently disabling condition usually treated medically but with unsatisfactory results for long-term relief with medical treatment alone.[2] However, back pain is a good example of how a coordinated, multidisciplinary, and comprehensive course of treatment produces the best chance of therapeutic gains. Pain Disorders are also costly in terms of the personal, social, occupational, educational, and financial areas of a patient's life.

BODY DYSMORPHIC DISORDER

Body Dysmorphic Disorder (BDD) is a puzzling disorder that produces substantial discomfort and dysfunction in patients and is difficult to treat. According to the *DSM-IV-TR*,[15] the diagnostic criteria include:

1. Preoccupation with an imagined defect in appearance or markedly excessive concern for a slight physical anomaly.
2. Preoccupation causes clinically significant distress or impairment in social, occupational, or other important areas of functioning.
3. Preoccupation is not better accounted for by another mental condition (e.g., Anorexia Nervosa, Obsessive-Compulsive Disorder).

Body Dysmorphic Disorder typically begins during adolescence and, although it occurs in both men and women, is slightly more common in women. Patients with BDD rarely self-refer to a mental health specialist and are rarely diagnosed by their primary care physician, so it difficult to accurately establish the number of BDD sufferers. This condition may appear abruptly or develop gradually and varies in intensity and persistence unless appropriately treated.[16]

Those with BDD are mostly concerned with the physical appearance of their head or face, sometimes the sexual organs, or other parts of their body, and obsession can shift from one part to another or involve several body parts at the same time. Concern may be of a general nature; for example, a well-developed man may think of himself as puny and try obsessively to gain weight, becoming a high risk for steroid abuse. Patients with Body Dysmorphic Disorder spend considerable time checking themselves and hours uncontrollably worrying about their appearance. Some continuously gaze at themselves in mirrors and others avoid mirrors. Most patients try to hide what they perceive as their deformity or try cosmetic surgery, although they are rarely satisfied with the results. They avoid going out to public places, including work and school, and avoid social situations, preferring to go out at night or not at all. Although the high levels of distress can lead to repeated hospitalizations and suicide attempts, patients are usually too embarrassed to seek help, and their condition could go undiagnosed for years. This condition clearly indicates much more than being unhappy with one's appearance; BDD is an obsession that consumes considerable time and money and produces significant distress.

Most patients with BDD will resist referrals to a mental health professional because they are convinced of the "reality" of their disfigurement, and they rarely follow through with suggested mental health treatments because they do not view their problem as a psychological issue. About 2 percent of people seeking corrective cosmetic surgery suffer from this condition,[30] the majority being women, but it is unclear whether this difference holds up in the general population.[2]

It is assumed that society's unrealistic expectations of what is attractive and exaggerated concerns for appearance are the basis for this disorder, although it is common for people who have Personality Disorders to frequently suffer from Body Dysmorphic Disorder as well. Some psychodynamic theorists have speculated about symbolic interpretations of the symptoms, but there is little evidence that these interpretations are valid.

In diagnosing BDD the therapist must first differentiate the obsessions from normal concerns about appearance and grooming and establish that significant distress and impaired functioning are present. Histrionic Personality Disorder will cause patients to obsess about their appearance, but these patients are usually trying to look better rather than trying to fix a perceived deformity.[2] In addition, valid medical problems must be ruled out as well as Mood and Anxiety Disorders, where negative self-image is evident. BDD may be confused with other conditions, including Schizophrenia, Social Phobia, and Obsessive-Compulsive Disorder, but if the symptoms are based on these conditions, then the diagnosis of BDD is not appropriate.

BDD is very difficult to treat, and the people who suffer from it sincerely believe that an aspect of their appearance is so grotesque and noticeable that no one could possibly disagree with them. They also feel that the only reason others do not agree with the assessment of their deformity is because they feel sorry for the person and are just trying to be nice. Some providers have found that selective serotonin reuptake inhibitor antidepressants are effective, while other antidepressant medications are not. One interpretation is that BDD is due, in part, to serotonergic dysregulation and may be linked to some type of Obsessive-Compulsive Disorder spectrum disorder. This is pure speculation with no real evidence, but it is an interesting hypothesis. A spectrum disorder is one that falls on a spectrum from a mild form of a disorder to more severe forms. Thus, people who think of BDD as a disorder on the Obsessive-Compulsive spectrum would argue that BDD is just a "type" of Obsessive-Compulsive Disorder.

Initially, treatment of BDD should begin, similarly to other Somatoform Disorders, by trying to discourage unnecessary medical procedures and surgeries that may leave the person feeling even more disfigured. Traditional insight-oriented psychotherapies have not proven effective, and the behavioral therapies and cognitive-behavioral therapy have yielded mixed results, although the use of cognitive-behavioral therapy is promising. Biological therapies like electroconvulsive therapy, antidepressant medications like tricyclics, andmonoamine oxidase inhibitors, and neuroleptic medications have also proven to be of little benefit. However, as mentioned above, selective serotonin reuptake inhibitors and clomipramine (serotonergic drugs) have produced some promising results, and it was reported that more than 50 percent of patients with BDD who were treated with one of these medications were significantly improved—more than would be expected if the same treatment was focused only on helping with the comorbid Depression.[31] Even though some treatments can be helpful to patients with BDD, patients usually do not get to an appropriate treating professional in a timely fashion. Patients with BDD seek help from their primary care physicians, plastic surgeons, dermatologists, or other specialists, but they do not seek mental health care unless referred by someone else.

Clearly, Body Dysmorphic Disorder is a complex condition, and it is important to educate patients and families as well as general medical providers and specialists (like plastic surgeons and dermatologists), about this condition and the treatments that are available. However, it is also clear that there is much more to learn about diagnosing and treating this challenging disorder.

OTHER TYPES OF SOMATOFORM DISORDERS

Undifferentiated Somatoform Disorder is a condition with one or more physical complaints (e.g., fatigue, loss of appetite, gastrointestinal or urinary symptoms) that cannot be fully explained medically or by the use of a drug. The symptoms must produce significant distress or impaired functioning lasting for at least six months and not intentionally produced. Because the condition cannot be better explained by another mental condition and lacks the specificity of the symptom patterns of the other Somatoform Disorders, it is called Undifferentiated Somatoform Disorder.

If a person suffers from some of the symptoms of Somatoform Disorder but not enough to be classified (even undifferentiated), then the diagnosis is Somatoform Disorder Not Otherwise Specified. This designation is rarely used and only if none of the other classifications are appropriate.

SUMMARY

Somatoform Disorders are the least understood psychological conditions, and yet the significant distress of psychological factors on physical functioning is now finally being recognized for the impact it has on families and society. We continue to learn more about how to categorize and diagnose these disorders, but we are still not treating them as effectively, medically or psychologically, as other classes and categories. We need more research, education, outreach, and prevention—more professional involvement at all levels—to offer better opportunities for treating these conditions and improving the lives of patients and their families.

11

Dissociative Disorders

Well, another invasion of the body snatchers event happened as usual, and Caroline took over tonight. Which is probably a good idea, because I was in no mood to handle anything. When Caroline and I changed places again tonight, Caroline imagined weaving her memories of the evening in with mine inside of our minds. It looked like she was weaving a ribbon in and out of my mind.

—Pilgram's Journey, Anonymous, 2010

BACKGROUND AND HISTORY

All of us can get lost in a good book or a movie, but someone with a Dissociative Disorder escapes reality in ways that are involuntary and unhealthy. Dissociative Disorders represent a class of psychiatric disorders that are characterized by a loss of control of the integration of identity, memory, and consciousness, usually as a result of a traumatic experience or multiple traumatic experiences. The symptoms range from amnesia to multiple identities and serve to repress the troublesome memories. Before the 19th century, people who displayed these types of symptoms were frequently accused of being possessed and were treated accordingly,[1] spawning reports of strange phenomena as well as an intense interest in spiritualism, parapsychology, and hypnosis. Many hypnotists discovered what appeared to be second personalities in some of their subjects and wondered how two minds could exist within one person.[2] A number of multiple personality cases emerged, which Rieber[3] estimated to be about 100, and, by the late 19th century, it was generally accepted that emotionally traumatic events could cause long-term psychological problems with a variety of symptoms.[4] Between 1880 and 1920, many international medical conferences addressed the issue of dissociation, and it was in this climate that Jean-Martin Charcot (with whom Freud studied) introduced his groundbreaking theories that a severe shock to the nervous system can cause a wide variety of neurological conditions. One of Charcot's students, Pierre Janet,[5] developed these ideas into a theory of dissociation, upon which Freud relied heavily in advancing his own theories.[6] Interest in dissociation waned in the early 20th century for a number of reasons, but one significant set of circumstances dealt a significant blow to this area of study. Following Charcot's death in 1893, many of his patients were exposed as frauds, and Janet's proposed theory was tarnished by his association with Charcot, and even Freud recanted his early emphasis on the importance of childhood trauma in dissociation.[2]

Although the medical and professional interest in these phenomena faded, public interest was very much alive in classical literature, with books such as Mary Shelley's *Frankenstein*, Robert Lewis Stevenson's *Strange Case of Dr. Jekyll and Mr. Hyde*, and many short stories by Edgar Alan Poe. This interest was also expressed in modern literature, movies, and television shows. In 1957 the book *The Three Faces of Eve* was published and later made into a movie, arousing the public's curiosity and resulting in a small but vocal group of clinicians who campaigned to make Multiple Personality a legitimate diagnosis.[7] Another highly influential book (and later a movie) titled *Sybil* was released in 1974, and it led to a significant resurgence of interest in Multiple Personality Disorder. Six years later, the diagnosis of Multiple Personality Disorder appeared in the *DSM-III*.[1]

As popular as this diagnosis is among the public, considerable controversy endures regarding the legitimacy of this condition. The fact that Multiple Personality Disorder is disproportionately found in North America gives some credence to the assumption that it is culturally bound and not truly a psychiatric condition. Others feel that it is a difficult condition to diagnose and, therefore, less sophisticated clinicians may not recognize the disorder when it is presented. Over the years, since the *DSM-III* introduced the formal diagnosis of Multiple Personality Disorder, mental health professions have modified how they view this condition, and, while many feel that it is a legitimate diagnosis, it is not as widely applied as it once was. Today, in the *DSM-IV-TR*, it is called Dissociative Identity Disorder (DID) and is diagnosed and treated as in the past, although the diagnostic criteria are more specific.

Dissociative Disorders are difficult to diagnose and treat, and therapists must use great care when dealing with patients who think they are suffering from Multiple Personality and avoid the power of suggestion that can complicate the case. For example, a woman was self-referred to me, had been in treatment for Multiple Personality Disorder with several other clinicians in the past, and presented with what she claimed were 16 different personalities (the exact number claimed by *Sybil*) and related an amazing (and difficult to believe) account about her childhood traumas. Her story, filled with inconsistencies, involved a worldwide conspiracy and events that were not consistent with reported history. First, it was important to decide whether this was a delusional system at work, multiple personality, fabrication, or symptoms of another disorder. After gently testing her beliefs, I believed that she did, in fact, think these events had happened to her, and yet it did not seem to be a true delusion. The history of her past therapies revealed a previous therapist who truly believed that she was a case of Multiple Personality and who had guided this patient through the discovery of past events that would explain the disorder. However, the discovered memories had no validation from anyone else in the family, were inconsistent with known elements in the person's history, did not fit any reported events in local history, and could not be validated in any way except from the hypotheses of the therapist, who claimed that the missing memories were due to lies, denial, and massive repression on the part of other people.

To approach treatment differently, a new, complex, and lengthy treatment plan was designed that carefully confronted the history of abuse and then integrated the different personalities (or ego states, as they are called) to resolve the Multiple Personality Disorder. Following two years of intense psychotherapy, the patient settled on a belief system that did not invalidate her history but gave her other interpretations to incorporate into her memories, and she was discharged with one personality and a feeling of optimism about her future.

This case clearly demonstrates the complexities of dealing with treating this type of diagnosis and the dangers of a patient desiring to meet the expectations of the therapist. Of course, most cases of Dissociative Identity Disorder are not quite so extreme and dramatic as the previous case, and often the different personalities or ego states are represented more subtly; this, too, is what makes them difficult to diagnose. Since everyone acts differently in different situations, it is not always easy to determine whether a person is manifesting different ego states or personalities or they are acting differently because of situational variance. When a person does present with different personality states, and they can be identified, then the job of dealing with the underlying trauma and integrating the personality can begin. While this is not usually as exciting or dramatic as portrayals in the media, it is a more typical example of the kinds of cases that are seen clinically.

DISSOCIATIVE DISORDERS IN GENERAL

Dissociative Disorders are disturbances in the organization of identity, memory, perception, or consciousness.[8] As originally described by Janet, dissociation may be best understood as disaggregation when events that are normally linked logically and temporally are isolated from other mental processes that would normally be working together.[5] The study of these phenomena led to Freud's theory of the subconscious[9] and Janet's[5] theory of dissociation, and these models are still used today to explain the phenomena of these conditions. The term *Dissociative Disorder* was introduced in 1980, when the *DSM-III* abandoned the term *hysteria* in favor of separate categories for Somatoform and Dissociative Disorders.[10]

Two broad types of memory can be referred to by different names: explicit and implicit,[11] declarative and procedural,[12] and episodic and semantic.[13] Explicit or episodic memory involves the recall of personal experiences identified with the self (I went to my son's basketball game last night). Implicit or procedural memory involves the execution of routine operations such as driving or typing. Episodic memory is primarily associated with limbic system functioning, primarily involving the hippocampal formation and mamillary bodies, and procedural memory appears to be a function of basal ganglia and cortical functioning.[14] It is suggested that different types of dissociative experiences are based, in part, on different memory systems.

In addition to the potential neurophysiological aspects of memory difficulties, there is compelling evidence that dissociation is linked with trauma[15] and that childhood physical or sexual abuse is linked with the development of dissociative symptoms.[16] Most theories of dissociation rely on the assumption that trauma is at the root of dissociation.

In terms of epidemiology, few valid studies exist on the frequency and distribution of Dissociative Disorders, although they are not a rare occurrence. Coons found that about 1 in 10,000 people in the general population suffer from dissociation, depending on the population studied.[17] Later research showed that Dissociative Disorders are probably more common than reported by Coons,[18] possibly as high as 1 percent of the population[19] and in specific populations (e.g., psychiatric patients) as high as 3 percent.[18] The majority of these patients are women; as high as 90 percent in some studies.[20] In one study, 110 patients admitted to a mental hospital (consecutively) were given a scale to assess dissociative experiences, and 15 percent of these patients scored high enough to meet the *DSM-III* criteria for Dissociative Disorder. Patients with high dissociative scores also had higher rates of Major Depression, Bipolar Disorder, Substance Abuse Disorders, and Borderline Personality Disorder. The researchers concluded that many more patients suffer from Dissociative Disorder than are usually identified.[21] The most common type of Dissociative Disorder in the United States is Dissociative Disorder NOS (Not Otherwise Specified),[21] and in other countries the dissociative trance and possession trance are the most common.[22]

When diagnosing any Dissociative Disorder, it is important to recognize that these are complex and often puzzling disorders that may be easily confused with other types of problems and conditions. Therefore, as in any other diagnosis, to make a diagnosis of a Dissociative Disorder, the symptoms must not be caused by another mental or physical disorder or be due to the effects of any drugs.[8]

DEPERSONALIZATION DISORDER

The essential feature of this Depersonalization Disorder (DPD) is the persistent feeling of unreality, detachment, or estrangement from oneself or one's body[23] and possibly perceiving a distortion of the size and shape of one's body or of other people and objects. Time seems to slow down, and the world may feel unreal, and these symptoms may last for a few moments or may come and go over many years.[24] Although these symptoms seem serious and can cause distress and impair functioning, they are not indicative of a Psychotic Disorder, and the person's reality testing remains intact. Commonly, depersonalization occurs with other symptoms such as anxiety, panic, or phobias, and these might be due to comorbid conditions, or perhaps they are symptoms that accompany the DPD. Depersonalization can be a symptom of Posttraumatic Stress Disorder (PTSD) but can also be related to alcohol or drug abuse or even as a side effect of prescription medications.[8] A similar symptom called derealization occurs when a person has an altered perception of her surroundings, which makes the world seem different or dreamlike. During these episodes, patients tend to ruminate anxiously and worry about their own mental and physical functioning, fearing that they are going crazy or are seriously ill.

Although depersonalization can be a very frightening experience, it is rarely serious by itself and will often remit spontaneously in a relatively short period of time. If this disorder occurs frequently or intensely, it may be a more complicated form of DPD or may be indicative of another disorder or syndrome. If it does not remit, brief treatment is usually effective, and self-hypnosis or relaxation can be helpful. Sometimes people are instructed to focus on the symptoms and to try to enjoy them; using techniques such as paradoxical intention (trying to produce or intensify the symptoms) the person can gain control of the process, make it less frightening, and have it disappear. Other successful forms of treatment for DPD are relaxation training and systematic desensitization, biofeedback, psychotherapy, and stress management. Medications are not typically useful in this condition unless they are used to treat comorbid conditions such as depression or anxiety.[8]

DISSOCIATIVE AMNESIA

Dissociative Amnesia (DA) involves significant memory loss that is more extensive than simple forgetfulness, and it cannot be explained by a physical or neurological condition. The most common type of amnesia is the absence from memory of traumatic events and periods, especially from childhood; the sudden-onset amnesia following a traumatic event, such as a motor vehicle accident, is rare.[24] It is a classic, functional disorder of episodic memory and does not involve procedural memory or problems with memory storage, and, unlike dementing illnesses, it is reversible.[5] The three main characteristics of DA are:

1. Memory loss is episodic (first-person things or events—what happened to you personally).
2. Memory loss is for one or more discrete time periods, ranging from minutes to years, and this involves a complete loss of memories encoded and stored. Unlike amnestic problems due to physical difficulties or injuries, there is no difficulty in retaining new episodic information, which means that amnesia in Dissociative Disorder is typically retrograde rather than anterograde,[25] although a few cases reported patients mimicking organic amnestic syndromes, which is having difficulty incorporating new information that mimics organic amnestic syndromes.[26]
3. Memory loss is usually due to traumatic or stressful events, and one study found that 60 percent of the studied cases involved child abuse.[16]

The diagnosis of DA is applied when the predominant disturbance is one or more episodes of inability to recall important personal information, usually of a traumatic or stressful nature, that is too extensive to be explained by ordinary forgetting. The symptoms must also cause significant distress and impair normal functioning.[27] Dissociative Amnesia frequently occurs following an episode of trauma; its onset may be gradual or sudden; it often occurs in the third and fourth decades of life;[28] and it usually involves one episode, although multiple episodes are not uncommon.[16] The memory loss is not vague or spotty but is rather a loss of any and all episodic memory for a finite period of time.[8] Although a person has no obvious memory for a particular episode or time period, he does seem to be aware of the world around him at some level. For example, a victim of assault or rape may not remember the event, but she may show other symptoms of trauma and act like a victim in other ways.[8] Further, amnesia victims typically do not have problems that involve their sense of identity.

Treatment for DA is often a matter of removing a person from the threatening situation and, as a result, may cause a spontaneous remission, which means that the person gets better on his own.[25] Victims of amnesia are often easily hypnotized and respond to techniques such as age regression as well.[29] Some people respond to the *screen technique*, a type of hypnosis where the person is asked to visualize the event as if it were projected onto a screen. This technique keeps the memory and affective response somewhat isolated[30] and might be used later with flashbacks if necessary. Psychotherapy with DA is fairly straightforward and involves trying to gain access to the dissociated memories, getting in touch with and working through the emotions associated with the memories, and then reintegrating these memories into the patient's conscious awareness. Treatment for this condition is usually very helpful and successful.[8]

DISSOCIATIVE FUGUE DISORDER (DFD)

Dissociative Fugue Disorder (DFD) resembles Dissociative Amnesia but with one major difference: the person actually puts real physical distance between herself and her real identity; this is called a *fugue state*. Occasionally, a story in the news features a person who has "come to" in a town or city different from where they live and has no idea where he is or how he got there. He may adopt a new identity and be capable of blending into the new environment. This state might last a few hours or, in rare cases, a few months, but the person will usually and abruptly snap out of it. When the person comes out of the fugue state, he is often disoriented, depressed, and angry, with no recall of recent events. Another difference between the DFD and DA is that, in the fugue state, the person forgets her true identity; with amnesia, that is rare.

There are cases of reported fugue episodes that are later determined to have been fabricated for some specific reason; thus, malingering must be considered and ruled out, especially if someone has something to gain or avoid by completely changing his circumstances. Fortunately, in the hands of an experienced clinician, malingering can usually be discovered, but it is sometimes difficult to determine.

Information on the epidemiology of the DFD is minimal, because it is a rare disorder, and it spontaneously remits in almost every case, meaning few people who experience it will seek treatment. Obviously, providing treatment for a condition that no longer exists is not a productive approach, and we typically do not hear about these situations unless they are on the news or in professional literature. A clinician will usually observe this unusual and interesting type of amnestic disorder after the person realizes her true identity, and at times people will seek treatment to understand what happened and to make sure they avoid similar episodes in the future. Because these events are often precipitated by stressful or traumatic situations, treatment usually focuses on dealing with the emotional aspects of the aftermath of the stressful or traumatic circumstances and then on reintegrating these emotions and events into the person's basic personality and memories. To accomplish this, the clinician will usually begin by reviewing the stressful or traumatic events that precipitated the fugue state and try to recover any lost memories about the episode.

DISSOCIATIVE TRANCE DISORDER

Dissociative phenomena have been described in virtually every culture,[31] and yet they are more prevalent in the less industrialized second- and third-world countries. Many cultures report numerous cases of people experiencing a dissociative trance state, although these occurrences are not frequently recognized and reported in more industrialized countries. In India, the one-year prevalence of Dissociative Trance Disorder is approximately 3.5 percent of all psychiatric hospitalizations, making it a common mental disorder in that culture.[22] Dissociative trance phenomena frequently involve sudden and extreme changes in sensory and motor control. In Latin American countries, an example of dissociative trance is the *ataque de nervios*, which has an estimated lifetime prevalence rate of 12 percent in Puerto Rico.[32] A typical episode of dissociative trance involves a sudden feeling of anxiety, followed by total body shaking that resembles convulsions, hyperventilation, unintelligible screaming, agitation, and violent body movements. Subsequent symptoms can involve collapse and a transient loss of consciousness, ending with fatigue and confusion when the episode is over. Many examples of dissociative trance phenomena are reported in different cultures.[8]

A similar phenomenon is a possession trance, which involves an assumption of a distinct alternative identity presumed to be that of a deity, ancestor, or spirit who has temporarily taken possession of the subject's mind and body. This is not the same condition as Dissociative Identity Disorder, in which the person has several distinct personalities or ego states within their personality. In a possession trance, the person feels that his personality has been overwhelmed or replaced with another entity. Treatments for this type of disorder depend on the culture but may involve rubbing the body with special potions, attempting to change the person's social circumstances, as well as physical restraint. It is also common to invoke certain ceremonies to appease the invading spirits and to drive them out or encourage them to abandon the possession.

DISSOCIATIVE IDENTITY DISORDER

Dissociative Identity Disorder involves the presence of two or more distinct personalities that represent very different ways of relating to other people and of perceiving the world around them. Historically, this fascinating and controversial disorder has been called Multiple Personality Disorder or Split Personality. The disorder is not related to Schizophrenia, although it is frequently confused with this condition in the media and is the subject of several books, movies, plays, and television shows. Historically, the term *schizophrenia* did not mean to infer that there is a split in a patient's personality or that multiple personalities or ego states develop. Rather, it explains that there is a split between cognition and affect, which means that a patient's thinking and emotions do not seem to fit together.

Although the entertainment media sometimes portray a character with an alternate personality being responsible for illegal or immoral acts (for example, Mr. Hyde), this is rarely the case.[33] The alternative personalities may be male or female, and each usually has a distinctly different way of talking, perceiving, and presenting him- or herself. DID can be found in children, although it is very rare; it usually emerges in teens and young adults. DID is rarely seen in people over the age of 40 and is found more frequently in women than in men. Typically, there is a significant gap between the emergence of symptoms and the formal diagnosis,[34] and, if untreated, this condition is chronic and recurrent and rarely remits spontaneously, although the symptoms may wax and wane.[8]

Transient dissociative episodes are a common and normative phenomenon during childhood and generally decrease during adolescence to a relatively low level in adulthood. However, pathological dissociation is a complex psychological process that results in a failure to integrate information into the normal stream of consciousness and results in a wide range of symptoms that are often misdiagnosed. Obviously, an accurate and timely diagnosis is important for a good prognosis.

A person with different identities will switch back and forth between them, particularly under stress. Patients often report feeling as though different people are living inside their head and who will talk and converse with each other. Each of these identities will have a name, personal history, and unique characteristics, including marked differences in manner, voice, gender, and physical qualities, such as the need for corrective eyewear. There are also differences between the personalities with respect to their awareness of the alternative ego states.[35]

No substantial evidence of DID exists, although some clinicians agree that the number of cases diagnosed in the United States and Europe has increased in the past few decades.[36] Some have estimated that there is a 1 percent incidence among psychiatric inpatients,[21] and some authors have suggested that the increase is due to social contagion, hypnotic suggestion, and misdiagnosis.[37] These patients tend to be highly suggestible and easily hypnotized, and care must be taken with the manner in which the disorder is discussed with them.[8] The recent increase in reported incidents may be attributed to frequent underreporting in the past. Common comorbidities include Depressive Disorders, Substance Use Disorders, and Borderline Personality Disorder. Some patients will exhibit or report other symptoms such as sexual, eating, and sleep difficulties;[8] some will describe somatic or conversion symptoms;[38] and others will experience psychosomatic symptoms such as migraine.[39]

Although most practitioners agree that DID is a legitimate diagnosis, it still remains controversial. For example, much of the attention, research, and writing about DID is in North America, with little discussion about it in other parts of the world. Some speculate that it is confined to North America and suggest that it is a culture-bound and iatrogenic (caused by the doctor) condition, although cases of this type appear to be on the decline.[40] Over the years, reports regarding the cases of "Eve" and "Sybil" gained much notoriety amid criticisms and questions about the validity of this diagnosis. Thigpen and Cleckley, who chronicled their treatment of Eve White in *The Three Faces of Eve*, later wrote about other people who had been diagnosed with DID, and the authors commented on the attraction to playing the multiple-personality role and the lengths to which some people will go to legitimize their self-diagnosis through a psychiatric authority. They observed that some patients "appear to be motivated (either consciously or unconsciously) by a desire to draw attention to themselves."[41] Certainly a diagnosis of Multiple Personality attracts more attention than most other diagnoses, and some patients appear to be motivated by secondary gain associated with avoiding responsibility for certain actions.[41] Several theories exist about the causes of DID, including that dissociative phenomena occur with other clinical disorders (e.g., other anxiety or depressive types of disorders) and various personality disorders (e.g., Histrionic or Borderline Personality Disorders), particularly when there is a history of trauma or abuse.[42] In comparison to other traumatized patients, DID patients reported severe and multifaceted traumas: physical and sexual trauma predicted somatoform dissociation, and sexual trauma predicted psychological dissociation. According to the memories of DID patients, the trauma occurred in an emotionally neglectful and abusive social context, and pathological dissociation was best predicted by early onset of reported intense, chronic, and multiple traumatization.[43]

In one interesting study, 98 women inpatients with a history of abuse completed self-report inventories for DID, PTSD, and other psychological problems. Of these, 83 percent reported dissociative symptoms that were greater than the median for normal adults, and 24 percent had scores at or above the median score for patients with PTSD. The researchers also found that patients with a history of childhood abuse reported higher levels of dissociative symptoms.[44]

Another theoretical approach suggests that neurochemical systems may be involved with DID and explain some of the memory loss experienced due to severe trauma. This implies that dissociation may be due in part to changes in the brain that may result from trauma or other phenomena. Similarly, Demitrack et al. studied 30 women with eating disorders and 30 women without eating disorders and found that the women with eating disorders had significantly higher levels of dissociative pathology.[45] They also found that the presence of severe dissociative experiences appeared to be specifically related to a propensity for self-mutilating and suicidal behavior. This study suggests that neurochemical systems, which are abnormal in patients with eating disorders, may be an underlying factor in some dissociative experiences. Other studies reported that neuropeptides, which are protein-like chemical messengers carrying information between cells, and neurotransmitters, which are chemicals released from neurons that directly affect adjacent neurons, may be involved in these types of disorders. When neuropeptides and neurotransmitters are released during stress, they can modulate memory function when acting at the level of the hippocampus, amygdala, and other brain regions that are related to memory. Such releases may interfere with the laying down of memory traces for incidents of childhood abuse and trauma and may result in long-term alterations in the function of the neuromodulators, a clear indication that extreme stress can have substantial impact on memory.[46]

The psychodynamic theorists focus more on the intrapsychic factors and how they might function under the effects of trauma and abuse. They emphasize the importance of psychological defenses like repression and denial in trying to understand dissociative phenomena. This approach assumes that when a person experiences severe abuse or trauma that is too difficult to deal with at a conscious level, the memory of it is repressed into the subconscious mind. Although the memory is not available to consciousness, it still might indirectly influence the person psychologically, such as by creating a distorted portrayal of the event. Trauma is the basis of dissociation, while psychological defenses alter the conscious manifestation of behavior, thoughts, and feelings associated with anything reminiscent of the trauma. According to psychodynamic theorists, dissociation is the manner in which the subconscious mind tries to protect the conscious mind from dealing with an event so traumatic that it would be devastating to think about it directly.

More recently, social psychologists theorize that dissociation occurs when people learn to enact the role of the multiple personality patient and to invoke alternative personalities as a means of expressing the thoughts and feelings they are incapable of experiencing and expressing directly when they are in their normal personality state. This social-psychological approach does not deny that long-standing attributes and cognitive styles may predispose someone to adopt this role more easily and convincingly than others, but they emphasize that the acquisition and portrayal of these roles is a learned process. Developing multiple identities is more involved than behaving as different people at different times. It requires reinterpreting the past in a manner that is consistent with the idea of possessing multiple selves. Typically, this involves attributing uncharacteristic, shameful, or disavowed aspects of earlier behavior to one or more alternative identities. DID may develop more readily in people who can actively and frequently imagine themselves in various roles handling situations differently than they ordinarily would. These fantasies can provide a fixed pattern and the basis for the emergence of new personalities who can consistently express things in ways that could not be done normally.[33]

All of the various theoretical approaches to DID are probably correct to some degree. This disorder is sometimes observed in ways that are not entirely consistent with the diagnostic criteria, which means that some people have some of the risk factors unique to DID but without manifesting enough of the diagnostic criteria to result in a formal diagnosis.

TREATMENTS FOR DISSOCIATIVE DISORDERS

Dissociative Disorders are a class of disorders characterized by a loss of control of the integration of identity, memory, and consciousness, usually occurring in the aftermath of single or multiple experiences of trauma. In general, the effective treatments include the psychotherapies that are designed to help patients work through traumatic memories and to control the access to the various dissociative states that have split off from the normal personality. Some clinicians have found that hypnosis can be helpful in some cases, and medications have value with some patients.[47] One exception to these general findings deals with Depersonalization Disorder, for which there appears to be no reliable and effective treatment, using either medication or psychotherapy. This disorder is characterized by a pervasive sense of unreality and detachment with intact reality testing, and therapy and medication do not seem to help. Typically, as mentioned above, this condition appears to be self-limiting and will usually resolve on its own. However, there is some evidence for dysregulation of endogenous opioid systems (parts of the brain that involve opioid-like chemicals such as endorphins, enkephalins, dynorphins, and endomorphins) in Depersonalization Disorder, and a few studies have suggested that opioid antagonists (drugs that block the opioid-like chemicals) may be effective in the treatment of dissociative or depersonalization symptoms.[48]

Some professionals have worked with patients to recover memories during therapy and find that doing so has a role in the treatment of Dissociative Disorders. They support the use of hypnosis as one way to explore the dissociative states in order to unlock some of the hidden or repressed memories.[49] This is a controversial area due to the unfortunate findings of the iatrogenic nature (symptoms caused by the treating professional) of some of the recovered memories and the outright fabrication of some of the findings. However, most clinicians can recall therapy sessions when a patient experienced a long repressed or forgotten event returning to consciousness, and there is evidence to support its validity. Issues of recovered memories must be considered carefully, neither denying nor unquestioningly embracing their existence. Knowing that some patients, and particularly DID patients, are highly suggestible makes it more likely that they may be led into believing that they have developed DID. The different roles they have used or fantasized may easily become alternative personalities.

Most of the literature on the treatment of Dissociative Disorders has focused on DID. Kluft points out that the treatment of DID patients resembles that of other traumatized populations and is stage oriented, with the first few stages being supportive and strengthening in nature.[50] While many find that medications are not of much help with DID or any of the Dissociative Disorders,[47] medication can make a significant difference in ameliorating severe and disabling symptoms that interfere with therapeutic progress.[51] The antidepressant medications (especially selective serotonin reuptake inhibitors) are the most helpful, because patients with DID often suffer from comorbid Depression. Anticonvulsants are sometimes helpful since there is a high comorbidity between DID and Seizure Disorders.[8]

Psychosocial treatments offer a number of ways to help patients with DID to gain control over the dissociative process.[52] It usually takes a long time for psychotherapy to work through the identities and to reintegrate them into the core personality, and some clinicians augment the therapy with hypnosis. Elements of the psychotherapy can involve introducing into consciousness some of the traumatic memories that led to the dissociation; this is usually a difficult process for the patient and must be done slowly and carefully. Dealing with DID in therapy can be a time-consuming and emotionally taxing process for both the patient and the therapist.

Schachter proposes a Rule of Thirds for treating DID[26]:

- Spend the first third of the psychotherapy session assessing the individual's current mental state and life problems and defining a problem area that might benefit from retrieval into consciousness a troubling memory and work through it.
- Spend the second third of the session accessing and working through this memory.
- Spend the final third helping the patient to assimilate the information, regulate and modulate emotional responses, and discuss any responses to the therapist that may seem to be related to the condition or the underlying trauma, as well as looking at plans for the immediate future with respect to the issues discussed.

The main goal of treatment for DID is the integration of the patient's multiple ego states (or personalities) and to help the patient feel whole, complete, and no longer fragmented. Some patients will resist because it is too threatening or they may not want to give up the protection and perceived benefits of the multiple identities.

SUMMARY

The Dissociative Disorders can be puzzling, frightening, difficult to diagnose, and challenging to treat. Although these disorders are often misunderstood or misjudged, we are developing better approaches to treating these conditions, and research is focusing on integrating the various theories and approaches that will, hopefully, set the course for future improvements. This is an area of theory and treatment that has a huge potential for some significant gains in the near future, and it appears that some substantial advances in our understanding and treatment of these conditions are near at hand.

12

Making Sense of It All

That the birds of worry and care fly over your head, this you cannot change, but that they build nests in your hair, this you can prevent.

—Chinese proverb

CHANGING CONCEPTIONS OF ANXIETY AND RELATED DISORDERS

The goal of this book is to provide a working definition for different types of Anxiety Disorders as well as useful explanations as to how they develop and are treated. I examine Somatoform and Dissociative Disorders in an effort to reveal the daily personal and social issues patients must face and to help others gain an appreciation for the subtlety and depth of these challenging disorders. All of us have experienced anxiety and moments when we briefly escape from reality through fantasy, media, or daydreaming; we have shared, albeit on a much smaller scale, the experiences of patients who suffer from these disorders, and yet most people will not cross that line into clinical pathology. To qualify for a formal or clinical diagnosis, specific and identifiable symptoms must create significant distress or interfere with daily normal functioning and must also exist over a particular period of time. Being diagnosed with one of these disorders requires much more than simply feeling anxious, obsessed or worried, and it is not always easy to understand the differences between normal functioning and true pathology.

There are many reasons why paying attention to these issues is important. Obviously, these disorders produce considerable misery in the people who suffer from them, and these problems usually have an impact on friends and family as well. Further, the formal and informal treatment of Anxiety and related disorders is a significant expense; however, the bigger expense comes in the form of lost work time and other indirect costs that are far more than the direct expenses associated with these disorders. Coping with symptoms of pain and suffering, usually without much respite, means that many or most routine tasks are a continuous struggle for these patients. Most of us will never experience feeling deathly afraid of something or being fearful of leaving home, but those with Anxiety Disorders may deal with these feelings daily.

Perhaps the most tragic aspect of Anxiety Disorders is that a large majority of patients do not have access to or receive the effective and appropriate treatments that are available. This uncomfortable fact is certainly true in underdeveloped regions of the world, but it is true in developed countries as well. Unfortunately, Anxiety and other related disorders do not generate public interest through telethons and major fund-raising programs for supporting research and treatment. It is important that we increase our attention and focus on the disease burden of mental health problems in the world as we do for other serious illnesses.

The progress of the past few decades, as a result of research in the treatment of Anxiety Disorders, is quite impressive. The recent gains made in the development of effective and safe medications for Anxiety Disorders are changing the lives of many patients, and I expect to see additional breakthroughs in the near future. However, medications will still serve primarily to control the symptoms of Anxiety Disorders and will not have a curative role. Likewise, it is unlikely that medications alone will provide the primary treatment breakthroughs for Somatoform and Dissociative Disorders, but I expect the continued development of new drugs that are more helpful and with fewer side effects.

There have been remarkable gains in the development and improvement of psychotherapeutic approaches to treatment, along with some evidence-based treatments that are clearly making a significant impact. However, the key to providing appropriate psychological treatment for these conditions lies in the hands of competent and trained professionals who can make a long-lasting difference in patients' lives. One of the challenges facing the mental health field is that, presently, there are not enough trained providers to help all the people who need treatment, especially those in rural and impoverished communities. It is embarrassing that our mental health treatment system has effective therapies available that could make a difference for many patients and their families, but they are not available because there are too few professional psychologists to meet the need, and most people do not even have a chance to get adequate treatment. I would suggest that this is not just a mental health problem but rather a public health and social problem that affects all of us.

In addition to medications, new and potentially valuable medical treatments are emerging that will likely change the approach to treating these disorders. Unique medical and surgical treatments will, in the near future, provide options that will result in entirely new ways of providing treatment, mostly in the area of relieving symptoms. Although they may not cure the specific disorder, these new treatments may return patients to a level of functioning that allows them a quality of life they may have never known before. Similarly, as we learn more about the potential role of genetics in establishing a predisposition for some of these disorders, a whole new world of treatment options opens up. Hopefully, someday, we will be able to genetically discover who might be at risk for certain conditions, such as Anxiety Disorders, and then modify the relevant genes to reduce the risk. These potential genetic treatments will not reduce the risk to zero, but by lessening the risk even a few percentage points, the potential benefits would be enormous. Breakthroughs in genetics, neurophysiology, neurochemistry, neuroimaging, as well as in psychology, psychopharmacology, and psychiatry will offer new treatment approaches we have yet to imagine.

The lack of access to appropriate treatment by many people—not just those in the underserved areas and developing countries—affects all mental health treatments. Since the early 1980s, insurers have controlled access to medical and mental health care, and the insurance companies have reduced the number of mental health visits as well as the circumstances under which a person is able to be seen. It is not uncommon to discover that an insurance company will only cover the services of certain providers and specific diagnoses and will deny coverage for chronic or preexisting conditions that do not meet their definition of *medical necessity*. The length of hospital stays beyond the first day are decided primarily by health insurance companies, and ill and suffering patients are often sent home with loved ones who are scared and do not have the skills or knowledge to handle the situation. Insurance almost never covers educational psychological testing and scholastic counseling; court-ordered testing and therapy in cases of divorce and custody disagreements; and rarely covers marital, family, or relationship counseling. Some insurance companies, including publicly funded ones such as Medicare and Medicaid, will not provide a list of participating providers to callers, which means that finding a mental health professional is the patient's responsibility; thus, patients must call office after office looking for someone who will accept them as a new patient. Medicaid used to offer a telephone number that patients could call and find a provider in their zip code area, but, due to budget cuts, this service has not been available for over a decade. Of course, many people cannot afford insurance premiums at any level or do not qualify for public assistance, and they simply go without care for all types of illnesses. These are people in our communities, our neighbors, our children's classmates, our coworkers, people in stores we frequent, and people on planes, trains, and buses we ride, and more of them every day are living without medical or mental health coverage of any sort. Clearly, the lack of adequate care for a large part of the population seriously affects all of us in our daily lives. Politicians repeatedly claim that they are trying to solve these problems, but in the past 30 years, little progress is evident.

One issue worth paying attention to is how thinking in the public, political, health and mental health arenas, and in the media, evolve and change over time. In the recent past, we talked about neuroses, and the treatment options were limited to a few pills and psychoanalytic psychotherapy, but now we classify these illnesses as Anxiety Disorders (as well as Somatoform and Dissociative Disorders), and treatment includes many therapeutic and medication choices. In reality, the types and availability of treatments depend more upon social factors than on medical or psychological ones. How society regards health, mental health, diagnosis, treatment, and other related factors determines how public and private funds are used to provide care and to decide who receives care and whether care is provided at all. Interestingly, one of the primary reasons for a lack of professional psychologists to provide needed care is the substantial decreases in funding for training programs, scholarships, and education—clearly, social and political choices. In general, people are more aware of and knowledgeable about mental health issues than they have been in the past, but the levels of ignorance, misinformation, bias, and stigma are still substantial and serious issues.

At this time, a new version of the Diagnostic and Statistical Manual is being prepared, the *DSM-V*. Research and progress dictate that probable changes will include the manner in which Anxiety and related disorders are classified and named. Most of the basic disorders will keep the same names; however, some of the criteria used to make a diagnosis will be changed. Presently, the *DSM-IV-TR* uses a prototypal approach, where each diagnosis requires a number of criteria from different categories of symptoms or signs. In the new *DSM-V*, disorders will likely be viewed dimensionally rather than categorically, and the diagnosis will depend on where someone falls within these dimensions rather than on the number of criteria a person has met.

The new classification scheme should reflect a better understanding of various conditions through the use of different words to label the diagnostic categories. This will probably occur in the Anxiety Disorders to some extent, but even more so in the Somatoform and Dissociative Disorders. The diagnoses of the latter two categories tend to be more vague, confusing, and controversial, since they have been formally recognized for fewer years than the Anxiety Disorders. Some of the Dissociative Disorders and are culture bound to some degree and will probably be modified in the *DSM-V*.

COPING WITH ANXIETY AND RELATED DISORDERS

Dealing with Anxiety Disorders involves improving prevention, treatment, coping strategies, education and training, and social and political action. For example, in most cases, Dissociative Disorders are notably related to trauma and abuse. Reducing the incidence and severity of these conditions is, without question, the best justification for implementing prevention through better education, improved reporting, and more responsive and timely treatment. Similarly, we need to educate both the public and medical providers about Somatoform Disorders, how they are manifested, and how they can be treated. Patients, too, need to understand that the diagnosis of a Somatoform Disorder is not a personal insult—this type of diagnosis does not mean that the physician or psychologist feels that it is "all in your head." It simply means that there is probably a psychological component to the real physical symptoms or concerns. Assuring patients that this diagnosis does not mean they are crazy or lying about their symptoms will help them to participate in and commit to a treatment plan.

Preventing or at least reducing the frequency of Anxiety Disorders also warrants our attention, and, again, education is the critical issue. Although most physicians will recognize and treat patients with anxiety, many are not familiar with the variety and availability of new and effective treatments. Mental health professionals should be responsible for sharing this information and for informing them of where they can refer patients for the care they need. In terms of preventing Anxiety Disorders, however, it is not so simple. Since the basis for many Anxiety Disorders is set during childhood, a disorder of this type usually involves early learning and even genetic predispositions, factors that cannot be changed easily, if at all. Certainly, we cannot modify a person's genetic endowment, although we may see in the not-too-distant future where this is possible. Similarly, we cannot change a person's history, but we can help people to learn from their past and to make changes today in ways that will help them to live healthier and happier lives. Treatment can also include learning to resist or recover from Anxiety Disorders that may have resulted from past events.

Minimizing and preventing Anxiety Disorders often relies heavily on a person's lifestyle, a person's ability to deal with stress and conflict, and her exposure to traumatic or stressful circumstances. Stress management is a critical aspect of preventing or minimizing anxiety. Therefore, a person will have a reasonable chance of avoiding Anxiety Disorders if he:

- gets enough sleep and rest
- exercises regularly
- has a healthy nutritional foundation
- does not smoke

- uses alcohol sparingly or not at all
- avoids recreational drugs such as marijuana and cocaine
- keeps stimulants (including coffee and caffeinated soda) to a minimum
- keeps a balanced lifestyle that includes recreation
- is appropriately socially active
- is productive at work or school but does not overdo or neglect other responsibilities
- takes good care of himself medically with regular physical exams
- follows doctors' orders
- seeks treatment when ill or injured
- avoids problematic activities such as excessive gambling
- effectively manages time
- does not overextend oneself financially or in terms of activities
- schedules time for relaxation and enjoyment

The problem for most of us is maintaining balance in our lives, and most of us have so much to do every day it is easy to feel trapped and unable to do anything about the many demands on our time. However, as soon as we allow ourselves to feel victimized by those things over which we have no control, we will often give up hope of ever having a normal life, and we have lost the battle.

While trying to help a particular patient gain a sense of control in her life, I encouraged her to take breaks at work and to make sure that she ate a nutritional lunch. This was a challenge for her, because she had discussed the fear of not having enough time in the day to take short breaks or a lunch period. I assured her that the research literature strongly supports the claim that people who to take regular breaks at work are more efficient and more productive, but it was a hard sell. Finally, she grew sick and tired of feeling sick and tired and began to take breaks during her work day. Very quickly she discovered that she was feeling better and accomplishing more, and her boss noticed and complimented her on taking better care of herself and on being a good role model for other employees—smart boss.

Frequently I hear the reverse argument from people who feel that it is impossible to make any reasonable changes in their lives and believe that they are completely trapped. They ask me to make them feel better but are unwilling to make any of the changes I suggest. Logically, of course, this makes no sense; how can someone expect to feel better when they are repeating the behaviors that are contributing to their feeling poorly? Members of Alcoholics Anonymous point to a quote from the Twelve-Step heritage: "If nothing changes—nothing changes." from a completely different arena, mathematical game theory offers an approach that is based on the idea of "win, stay—lose, change." In other words, if what you are doing produces the outcomes that you desire, then continue to do it; on the other hand, if what you are doing leads to undesirable outcomes, then stop and do something different. The goal of treatment is usually to help the patient discover new ways of dealing with her concerns in order to realize better outcomes, but it also means that the patient must be receptive to a different way of thinking and of doing things that will help her.

Exercising daily is a relatively simple task that is enormously helpful in dealing with mental health conditions, especially Anxiety and Mood Disorders. Yet I frequently hear from patients that they have no time for it. Consider for a moment how a busy person will always find the time to add one more meeting or one more errand into their already crowded schedule. Each of us needs to identify blocks of time for taking care of ourselves *before* we fall victim to everyone else's scheduling needs. One's own good health must be a daily priority; others will respect such efforts, and it will be easier to consider making other necessary changes when you have better control of your time.

Dealing with and preventing Anxiety and other related disorders boils down to two words: *balance* and *assertiveness*. Maintaining a well-balanced life means meeting one's responsibilities along with enjoying periods of relaxation, rest, recreation, exercise, and socialization. To achieve all of the above, efficiency is necessary. Efficiency means making the best use of blocks of time but not allowing oneself to become trapped in a routine that feels like a hamster running full tilt on a wheel. It is okay, occasionally, to set aside a chore in order to take a walk with a spouse or throw a ball to a child or just sit and read for 15 minutes.

Efficiency also means avoiding time wasters, such as television and video games, a trap for many. Picking a few enjoyable shows to watch per week or playing a game for a short, finite period of time is different from sitting for hours each day channel surfing, watching programs, and hanging onto a game remote just to kill time. Also, a couch potato usually combines mindless viewing with eating junk food and drinking soda or alcohol, all of which have a significant negative impact on health. It is frightening to read studies reporting that many children spend four to seven hours *per day* watching TV or playing video games. This means that the majority of their life, outside of school and sleeping, is spent in front of some form of electronic entertainment. It is essential, therefore, to make watching TV or playing video games a conscious choice rather than a default activity. I constantly remind parents to place—and enforce—time limits on TV and video games both for themselves and for their children. No child's life has ever been ruined because they had to stop playing "Call of Duty" before they wanted to. Toddlers need quiet time to engage their imaginations and create stories with their toys and should not have a continuous droning of television audio in the background. They need to develop skills such as focusing and concentrating on the activity in which they are engaged rather than be continuously interrupted by random noises.

Assertiveness, in U.S. culture, is often confused with aggressiveness. Being aggressive means acting in a way that will directly negatively impact or hurt or establish dominance over another person. Being assertive, on the other hand, means behaving in a manner that ensures your needs are being met, but not at the expense of another person. I tell my patients that assertiveness simply means acting in ways that convey to others: "My needs are just as important as your needs; not more important, but not less important either." Women patients tend to report that they feel as if everyone else's needs must be met before they can do anything for themselves, which, of course, includes their children, spouse, partner, parents, and so on. It is neither reasonable nor possible to completely meet everyone else's needs and expectations, and is important to understand that you will do a better job of taking care of others if you take care of yourself first. This is not being selfish; it is just a reality. Further, by assertively taking care of yourself you are modeling for others, including your children, how to avoid unhealthy patterns that define most people's lives and maintain a balance that ensures we do the essential tasks and still have time for the fun.

BEING A POSITIVE VOICE FOR GOOD MENTAL HEALTH

The best way to be a positive voice for mental health is to be a good role model; doing the things that are necessary to keep yourself physically and mentally healthy is the loudest voice of all. One challenge to making healthy and productive changes in one's life is that the old dysfunctional patterns are deeply ingrained habits and are not easy to change. Making small but consistent steps and sticking to them is the best method; small changes begin to mount up until major changes have occurred, and after awhile it becomes second nature. Too often people try to do too much at once, and when they are not successful at everything, they just give up.

Speaking out publicly for mental health is also important, and there are numerous ways of accomplishing this in a positive and constructive manner. Writing to politicians and voting are good ways to exert influence, but these actions can be frustrating as well. Politicians' vague responses typically reflect the latest polls and include a reassuring message, basically telling constituents what they want to hear. A more effective tactic is to watch how politicians vote on issues concerning mental health legislation and actively work to elect someone else if they do not vote the way you would like. When you contact politicians, it is important to let them know that you are a constituent and express your interests and preferences. Regardless of what they say, most politicians are primarily interested in being re-elected. If you and others voice your concerns clearly on how you feel about certain issues, they will pay attention, and the sooner you will see positive change. For example, in New York State, many concerned professionals, politicians, and citizens worked hard to enact legislation to ensure mental health parity, which means that patients could not be discriminated against just because they have a mental health problem. Insurers cannot charge different copayments for mental health visits, cannot artificially limit the number of visits, and must treat mental health coverage just like medical coverage. Even though there was substantial research from independent sources that proved that mental health parity did not drive up costs, there was huge opposition from the insurance and managed care industries, and it was a difficult struggle for many years before this legislation (known as Timothy's Law in New York) was passed. Not surprisingly, the final bill was watered down to get it passed, but it was enacted, and concerned parties continue to work to make the law even better. This was a good example of how people can work together to make changes happen. It was not an easy task but certainly was a cause worth fighting for.

In addition to contacting politicians, the message for good mental health programs and practices must be carried to schools, hospitals, and mental health facilities and programs. Teachers and school administrators wield considerable influence over children for a substantial portion of most days in the year. Encouraging schools to support positive mental health through nutrition and public health education, good psychoeducational and psychosocial programs, and appropriate staffing is essential for good public health in our communities. Programs such as sports, music, drama, clubs, and outreach all help children to become healthy, happy, and productive adults.

Mental health is closely aligned with physical health, which is largely dependent on diet and on the ability to exercise and enjoy sports and other activities. For the past two decades, childhood obesity has become a national epidemic, and insisting that all schools offer nutritious menu choices of low-fat, high-fiber foods and eliminating soda and candy machines from schools is a place to start. Having healthy food choices and good health practices in our own homes is also an important message to our children. Retaining physical education as part of the school curriculum not only gives students opportunities for physical activity, but it teaches them that daily exercise is important to stay active and healthy. Learning lifelong sports, such as tennis, cross-country skiing, basketball, volleyball, running/jogging, and bowling, is a way to convey to children that it is possible and necessary to exercise as adults, even in to the senior years. Similarly, learning to appreciate and participate in the fine arts, such as playing a musical instrument, chorus, dancing, sculpting, painting, and drawing, as well as learning to use technologies in the arts is also essential for a civilized and productive society. Businesses today are crying out for new ideas and employees who can creatively solve problems and generate innovative solutions. People who are broadly and liberally educated in a variety of areas are the future employees, scientists, teachers, and professionals that the world needs.

Another way to improve mental and social health in schools and society is to address the problems of physical and verbal abuse. Bullying in the schools, in the workplace, at home, and in public is finally being recognized for what it is: physical or verbal abusive behavior toward someone who cannot defend themselves. The more children and adults are held accountable for their behavior and feel that there is an avenue of recourse should they feel threatened or intimidated, the fewer stress-related absences there will be in schools and businesses. Organizations that are recognizing and dealing with these types of problems are showing the kinds of awareness and leadership that will help prevent some of the mental health problems of the future.

We can also be a positive influence in the workplace by making it a healthier and more productive part of our lives. Too often, businesses ignore the people side of the workplace, considering it a waste of time and money. Research convincingly demonstrates, however, that companies and organizations that take care of their employees are able to recruit and keep the best employees, who in turn are more productive and satisfied with their jobs. Programs through the American Psychological Association and various state psychological associations support and annually recognize companies for having a psychologically healthy workplace and encourage policies that reduce stress and create a pleasant work environment. This is sometimes a hard sell to executives, and especially to those who say things like, "This is a tough business, and if an employee isn't tough enough to handle the job, then let them find another place to work." This sounds very Darwinian and almost makes sense, except that when an organization creates a stressful work environment, it will certainly lead to increased voluntary turnover. Executives and administrators should keep in mind that when voluntary turnover escalates, it is often the best employees who leave first because they are good enough to find a job elsewhere, and those who are underproducing or not doing their jobs are the ones likely left behind.

Money spent to create a healthy work environment more than pays for itself in reduced turnover, higher productivity, and lower levels of absenteeism. Examples of meeting the human needs of employees might include benefits such as on-site day care for children of employees; maternity, paternity, and adoption leave; education benefits (paid time off to take classes or tuition reimbursement); training programs; health-related programs on site (e.g., exercise, smoking cessation groups, weight loss programs, and stress management); an employee assistance program, and a wellness center on site. Although these programs may cost money, they usually turn out to be cost effective in the long run; this is not just good treatment of employees—this is good business.

MAKING A DIFFERENCE

Educating ourselves about issues of health and mental health, including Anxiety and related disorders, is a place to start. Relying again on wisdom from the Twelve-Step heritage, we have to "talk the talk," but, even more importantly, we have to "walk the walk." Educating others about the Anxiety Disorder a family member or friend is dealing with is much more effective than simply complaining about how insensitive and ignorant people can be. If we truly want to make a difference, then we must also reach out and help others who may not be able to help themselves. This could include speaking with people who have similar conditions, getting involved with a self-help group, or even volunteering to give a speech to a group that would like to learn more about these disorders. Helping others is often a very good way to help ourselves, and we should always be on the alert for opportunities to do both.

The message that I would like to leave with readers is: "We are only helpless if we allow ourselves to be." Bad and unfortunate events will happen to all of us at one time or another, but assuming the role of victim is a choice, and one we should avoid. The role of victim traps us in situations where we feel passive and helpless, but taking responsibility for our own choices and health, as well as helping and supporting others to take control of their own lives, can result in our being a positive influence in our families and communities.

Resources

ORGANIZATIONS

American Psychiatric Association
1000 Wilson Boulevard, Suite 1825
Arlington, VA 22209-3901
703-907-7300/888-35-PSYCH
www.heathyminds.org

American Psychological Association
750 First Street, NE
Washington, DC 20002-4242
800-374-2721/202-336-5500
www.apa.org

Anxiety Disorders Association of America
8730 Georgia Avenue, Suite 600
Silver Spring, MD 20910
240-485-1001
www.adaa.org

National Alliance on Mental Illness
Colonial Place Three
2107 Wilson Boulevard, Suite 300
Arlington, VA 22201-3042
703-542-7600/800-950-6264
www.nami.org

National Institute of Mental Health
Science Writing, Press, and Dissemination Branch
6001 Executive Boulevard

Room 8184, MSC 9663
Bethesda, MD 20892-9663
866-615-6464/301-443-4513
www.nimh.nih.org

National Mental Health Association
2001 Beauregard Street, 6th Floor
Alexandria, VA 22311
800-969-NMHA/703-684-7722
www.nmha.org

WEBSITES

Anxiety Centre. "Famous People Affected by an Anxiety Disorder" (2010), www
.anxietycentre.com/anxiety-famous-people.shtml.
Healthy Place. "Anxiety in the Elderly" (2007), http://www.healthyplace.com/anxi
ety-panic/main/anxiety-in-the-elderly.html.
Healthy Place. "Mental Health Problems among Minorities" (2002), http://www
.healthyplace.com/anxiety-panic/main/mental-health-problems-among-
minorities.
Healthy Place. "Women and Anxiety: Twice as Vulnerable as Men" (2007), http://
www.healthyplace.com/anxiety-panic/main/women-and-anxiety.html.
Mayo Clinic. "Dissociative Disorders" (2009), http://www.mayoclinic.com/health/
dissociative-disorders/DS00574/DSECTION=symptoms.
Phillips, K. A. "Somatization Disorder" (2008), http://www.merck.com/mmhe/print/
sec07/ch099/ch009e.html.
Psychiatry.HealthSE.com. "Generalized Anxiety Disorder (GAD)." *Current Medical
Diagnosis & Treatment in Psychiatry* (2005), http://psychiatry.healthse.com/psy/
more/generalised_anxiety_disorder_gad/.
Psychiatry.HealthSE.com. "Panic Disorder and Agoraphobia." *Current Medical Diagnosis & Treatment in Psychiatry* (2005), http://psychiatry.healthse.com/psy/
more/panic_disorder_and_agoraphobia/.
Psychiatry.HealthSE.com. "Post-Traumatic Stress Disorder (PTSD)." *Current Medical
Diagnosis & Treatment in Psychiatry* (2005), http://psychiatry.healthse.com/psy/
more/post_traumatic_stress_disorder_ptsd/
University of Maryland Medical Center. "Anxiety Disorders." *Medical References; Patient Education* (2008), http://www.umn.edu/patiented/articles/what_anxiety_
disorders_000028-1.htm.
Yates, William R. "Somatoform Disorders" (2008), http://emedicine.medscape.com/
article/294908-print.

BOOKS AND ARTICLES

American College of Obstetricians and Gynecologists. "ACOG Practice Bulletin:
Use of Psychiatric Medications during Pregnancy and Lactation." *Obstetrics
and Gynecology* 111, no. 4 (2008): 1001–1020.

American Psychiatric Association. *Diagnostic and Statistical Manual, Fourth Edition, Text Revision*. Washington, DC: American Psychiatric Association, 2000.

Antony, M. M., and R. P. Swinson. *Phobic Disorders and Panic in Adults: A Guide to Assessment and Treatment*. Washington, DC: American Psychological Association, 2000.

Antony, M. M., and M. B. Stein, eds. *Handbook of Anxiety and Related Disorders*. New York: Oxford University Press, 2009.

Bandura, A. *Principles of Behavior Modification*. New York: Holt, Rinehart, & Winston, 1969.

Barlow, D. H. *Anxiety and Its Disorders: The Nature and Treatment of Anxiety and Panic*. 2nd ed. New York: Guilford Press, 2002.

Barlow, D. H., ed. *Clinical Handbook of Psychological Disorders*. New York: Guilford Press, 1993.

Beck, A. T., and G. Emery. *Anxiety Disorders and Phobias: A Cognitive Perspective*. New York: Basic Books, 1985.

Brawman-Mintzer, O., and R. B. Lydiard. "Psychopharmacology of Anxiety Disorders." *Psychiatric Clinics of North America* 1 (1994): 51–79.

Breuer, J., and S. Freud. "Studies on Hysteria." In *The Standard Edition of the Complete Psychological Works of Sigmund Freud*, edited by J. Strachy (trans. ed.). London: Hogarth Press (originally published in 1893–1895), 1955.

Eysenck, H. J., ed. *The Biological Basis of Personality*. Springfield, IL: Charles C. Thomas, 1967.

First, M. B., and A. Tasman. *DSM-IV-TR Mental Disorders: Diagnosis, Etiology, and Treatment*. Hoboken, NJ: John Wiley, 2004.

Freud, S. *New Introductory Lectures in Psychoanalysis*. Edited by James Strachey, *The Complete Works of Sigmund Freud*. New York: W. W. Norton, 1965.

Gabbard, G. O., ed. *Treatment of Psychiatric Disorders*, 3rd ed. Washington, DC: American Psychiatric Publishing, 2001.

Kagan, J., J. S. Reznick, and N. Snidman. "Biological Bases of Childhood Shyness." *Science* 240, (1988): 167–71.

Mowrer, O. H. "Stimulus Response Theory of Anxiety." *Psychological Review* 46 (1939): 553–65.

National Institute of Mental Health. *Anxiety Disorders*. Washington, DC: National Institute of Mental Health, 2009.

Putnam, F. W. *Diagnosis and Treatment of Multiple Personality Disorder*. New York: Guilford Press, 1989.

Rachman, S. *Fear and Courage*, 2nd ed. New York: Freeman, 1990.

Rogers, C. R. *On Becoming a Person*. New York: Houghton Mifflin, 1961.

Sadock, B., and V. Sadock. *Comprehensive Textbook of Psychiatry*, 7th ed. Philadelphia: Lippincott, Williams & Wilkins, 2000.

Sadock, B., and V. Sadock. *Kaplan and Sadock's Synopsis of Psychiatry: Behavioral Sciences/Clinical Psychiatry*, 9th ed. Philadelphia: Lippincott, Williams, & Wilkins, 2002.

Swartz, Karen L. *The Johns Hopkins White Papers*. Baltimore: Johns Hopkins Medical School, 2007.

Swartz, K. L. *The Johns Hopkins White Papers*. Baltimore: Johns Hopkins Medical School, 2008.

Watson, J. B., and R. Rayner. "Conditional Emotional Reactions." *Journal of Experimental Psychology* 3 (1920): 1–14.

References

CHAPTER 1

1. University of Maryland Medical Center. "Anxiety Disorders." *Medical References; Patient Education* (2008). http://www.umm.edu/patiented/articles/what_anxiety_disorders_000028-1.htm.

2. Swartz, Karen I. "Depression and Anxiety." In *The Johns Hopkins White Papers*. Baltimore: Johns Hopkins Medical School, 2007.

3. Freud, Sigmund. *New Introductory Lectures in Psychoanalysis*. Edited and translated by James Strachey, *The Complete Works of Sigmund Freud*. New York: W. W. Norton, 1965.

4. Twenge, Jean M. "The Age of Anxiety? Birth Cohort Change in Anxiety and Neuroticism, 1952–1993." *Journal of Personality and Social Psychology* 79, no. 6 (2000): 1007–21.

5. Clark, L. A., and D. Watson, "Tripartite Model of Anxiety and Depression: Psychometric Evidence and Taxonomic Implications." *Journal of Abnormal Psychology* 100, no. 3 (1991): 316–36.

6. Anxiety Centre. "Famous People Affected by an Anxiety Disorder" (2010). www.anxietycentre.com/anxiety-famous-people.shtml.

CHAPTER 3

1. Dupont, R. L., D. P. Rice, L. S. Miller, S. S. Sharaki, C. R. Rowland, and H. J. Harwood. "Economic Costs of Anxiety Disorders." *Anxiety* 2, no. 4 (1996): 167–72.

2. Psychiatry.HealthSE.com. "Panic Disorder and Agoraphobia." *Current Medical Diagnosis & Treatment in Psychiatry* (2005), http://psychiatry.healthse.com/psy/more/panic_disorder_and_agoraphobia/.

3. Greenberg, P. E., T. Sisitsky, R. C. Kessler, S. T. Finkelstein, E. R. Berndt, J.R.T. Davidson, J. C. Ballenger, and A. J. Fyer. "The Economic Burden of Anxiety Disorders in the 1990s." *Journal of Clinical Psychiatry* 60 (1999): 427–35.

4. Lowe, Patricia A. "Does a Relationship Exist between Gender and Anxiety across the Life Span?" Paper presented at the Annual Meeting of the National Association of School Psychologists (Proceedings). Toronto, Canada, 2003.

5. Brenes, Gretchen A., Jack M. Guralnik, Jeff D. Williamson, Linda P. Fried, Crystal Simpson, Eleanor M. Simonsick, and Brenda W.J.H. Pennix. "The Influence of Anxiety on the Profession of Disability." *Journal of the American Geriatrics Society* 53 (2005): 34–39.

6. Healthy Place. "Women and Anxiety: Twice as Vulnerable as Men." (2007), http://www.healthyplace.com/anxiety-panic/main/women-and-anxiety.html.

7. Patel, Vikram. "Gender and Mental Health Research in Developing Countries." Paper presented at the Global Forum for Health Research (Proceedings, p. 9). Arusha, Tanzania, 2002.

8. Cox, B.J., R.P. Swinson, I.D. Shulman, K. Kuch, and J.T. Reichman. "Gender Effects and Alcohol Use in Panic Disorder with Agoraphobia." *Behavioral Research and Therapy* 31 (1993): 413–16.

9. Yonkers, K.A., C. Zlotnick, J. Allwsorth, M. Warshaw, T. Shea, and M.B. Keller. "Is the Course of Panic Disorder the Same in Women and Men?" *American Journal of Psychiatry* 155 (1998): 596–602.

10. Diala, C. C., and C. Muntaner. "Mood and Anxiety Disorders among Rural, Urban, and Metropolitan Residents in the United States." *Community Mental Health Journal* 39, no. 3 (2003): 239–52.

11. Creamer, M., and R. Parslow. "Trauma Exposure and Posttraumatic Stress Disorder in the Elderly: A Community Prevalence Study." *American Journal of Geriatric Psychiatry* 16, no. 10 (1008): 853–56.

12. Nydegger, R.V., L.A. Nydegger, and F. Basile. "PTSD and Coping in Career Professional Firefighters." Paper presented at the International Business and Economic Research Conference, Las Vegas, Nevada, October 2010.

13. American Psychiatric Association. *Diagnostic and Statistical Manual, Fourth Edition, Text Revision.* Washington, DC: American Psychiatric Association, 2000.

14. Lavigne, J.V. "The Prevalence of ADHD, ODD, Depression, and Anxiety in a Community Sample of 4-Year-Olds." *Clinical Child and Adolescent Psychology* 38, (2009): 315–28.

15. First, M.B., and A. Tasman. *DSM-IV-TR Mental Disorders: Diagnosis, Etiology, and Treatment.* Hoboken, NJ: John Wiley, 2004.

16. Straus, C.C., and C.G. Last. "Social and Simple Phobias in Children." *Journal of Anxiety Disorders* 7 (1993): 141–52.

17. Anderson, J.C., S. Williams, R. McGee, and P.A. Silva. "DSM-III Disorders in Preadolescent Children." *Archives of General Psychiatry* 44 (1987): 69–76.

18. Last, C.G., S. Perrin, M. Hersen, and A.E. Kazdin. "A Prospective Study of Childhood Anxiety Disorders." *Journal of the American Academy of Child and Adolescent Psychiatry* 35 (1996): 1502–10.

19. Ginsburg, G., M. Riddle, and M. Davies. "Somatic Symptoms in Children and Adolescents with Anxiety Disorders." *Journal of the American Academy of Child and Adolescent Psychiatry* 45, no. 10 (2006): 1179–87.

20. Allen, J.L., and R.M. Rapee. "Are Reported Differences in the Events for Anxious Children and Controls Due to Comorbid Disorders?" *Journal of Anxiety Disorders* 23, no. 4 (2009): 511–18.

21. Roberts, R.E., C.R. Roberts, and W. Chan. "One-Year Incidence of Psychiatric Disorders and Associated Risk Factors among Adolescents in the Community." *Journal of Child Psychology and Psychiatry* 50, no. 4 (2009): 405–15.

22. Chen, H., P. Cohen, J. Johnson, and S. Kasen. "Psychiatric Disorders during Adolescence and Relationships with Peers from Age 17 to Age 27." *Social Psychiatry and Psychiatric Epidemiology* 44, no. 3 (2009): 223–30.

23. Ginsburg, G., and K.L. Drake. "Anxiety Sensitivity and Panic Attach Symptomatology among Low-Income African-American Adolescents." *Journal of Anxiety Disorders* 16, no. 1 (2002): 83–96.

24. Lowry, Kirsten A. "Interpersonal Problems, Adult Attachment, and Emotional Regulation among College Students with Generalized Anxiety Disorder, Panic Disorder, and Social Phobia." Working Paper, University of Nevada, Reno, 2009.

25. Ollendick, T.H., M.A. Jarrett, A.E. Grills-Taquechel, L.D. Hovey, and J.C. Wolff. "Comorbidity as a Predictor and Moderator of Treatment Outcome in Youth with Anxiety, Affective, Attention Deficit/Hyperactivity Disorder, and Opposition/Conduct Disorders." *Clinical Psychology Review* 28, no. 8 (2008): 1447–71.

26. Alfano, C.A. "Sleep-Related Problems among Children and Adolescents with Anxiety Disorders." *Journal of the American Academy of Child and Adolescent Psychiatry* 46, (2007): 224–32.

27. Kimel, L.K. "Phenomenology of Anxiety and Fears in Clinically Anxious Children with Autistic Spectrum Disorders." Working Paper, University of Denver, 2009.

28. Emslie, G.J. "Pediatric Anxiety—Underrecognized and Undertreated." *New England Journal of Medicine* 359, no. 26 (2008): 2835–36.

29. Jorm, A.F., A.J. Morgan, and A. Wright. "Interventions That Are Helpful for Depression and Anxiety in Young People: A Comparison of Clinicians' Beliefs with Those of Youth and Their Parents." *Journal of Affective Disorders* 111, no. 2–3 (2008): 227–34.

30. Ginsburg, G.S. "The Child Anxiety Prevention Study: Intervention Model and Primary Outcomes." *Journal of Consulting and Clinical Psychology* 77, no. 3 (2009): 580–87.

31. Brenes, G.A. "Age Differences in the Presentation of Anxiety." *Aging and Mental Health* 10, no. 3 (2006): 298–302.

32. Brenes, G.A., M. Knudson, W.V. McCall, J.D. Williamson, M.E. Miller, and M.A. Stanley. "Age and Racial Differences in the Presentation and Treatment of Generalized Anxiety Disorder in Primary Care." *Journal of Anxiety Disorders* 22, no. 7 (2008): 1128–36.

33. DeBeurs, E., A.T.F. Beekman, A.J.L.M. Van Baldom, D.J.H. Deeg, R. van Dyck, and W. van Tilburg. "Consequences of Anxiety in Older Persons: Its Effect on Disability, Well-Being and Use of Health Services." *Psychological Medicine* 29, (1999): 583–93.

34. Beekman, A.T.F., M.A. Bremmer, D.J.H. Deeg, A.J.L.M. Van Balkom, J.J. Smit, E. De Beurs, R. Van Dyck, and W. Van Tilburg. "Anxiety Disorders in Later Life: A Report from the Longitudinal Aging Study Amsterdam." *International Journal of Geriatric Psychiatry* 13, no. 10 (1999): 717–26.

35. DeBeurs, E., A.T.F. Beekman, D.J.H. Deeg, R. Van Dyck, and W. Van Tilburg. "Predictors of Change in Anxiety Symptoms of Older Persons: Results from the Longitudinal Aging Study Amsterdam." *Psychological Medicine* 30 (2000): 515–27.

36. "Treating Generalized Anxiety Disorder in the Elderly." *Harvard Mental Health Letter*. Boston: Harvard Medical School, 2009.

37. Roy-Byrne, P.P., M.G. Craske, M.B. Stein, G. Sullivan, A. Bystritsky, W. Katon, D. Golinelli, and C.D. Sherbourne. "A Randomized Effectiveness Trial of Cognitive-Behavioral Therapy and Medication for Primary Care Panic Disorder." *Archives of General Psychiatry* 62 (2005): 290–98.

38. Ivera, J., S. Benavarre, M. Rodriguez, T. Lorente, C. Pelegrin, J.M. Calvo, J.M. Leris, D. Idanez, and S. Amal. "Prevalence of Psychiatric Symptoms and Mental Disorders Detected in Primary Care in an Elderly Spanish Population. The Psicotard Study: Preliminary Findings." *International Journal of Geriatric Psychiatry* 23, no. 9 (2008): 915–21.

39. Sue, D.W. "Culture-Specific Strategies in Counseling: A Conceptual Framework." *Professional Psychology: Research and Practice* 21 (1990): 424–33.

40. Healthy Place. "Mental Health Problems among Minorities." *HealthyPlace. com* (2002), http://www.healthyplace.com/anxiety-panic/main/mental-health-problems-among-minorities.

41. Brown, C., M.K. Shear, H.C. Schulberg, and M.J. Madonia. "Anxiety Disorders among African-American and White Primary Medical Care Patients." *Psychiatric Services* 50, (1999): 407–9.

42. Brown, D.R., W.W. Eaton, and L. Sussman. "Racial Differences in Prevalence of Phobic Disorders." *Journal of Nervous and Mental Disease* 178, no. 7 (1990): 434–41.

43. Friedman, S., and C. Paradis. "Panic Disorder in African Americans: Symptomatology and Isolated Sleep Paralysis." *Culture, Medicine and Psychiatry* 28, no. 2 (2002): 179–96.

44. Arean, P.A., L. Ayalon, C. Jin, C.E. McCullock, K. Linkins, H. Chen, B. McDonnell-Herr, S. Levkoff, and C. Estes. "Integrated Specialty Mental Health Care among Older Minorities Improves Access but Not Outcomes: Results of the Prime Study." *International Journal of Geriatric Psychiatry* 23, no. 10 (2008): 1086–92.

45. Iwamasa, G.Y., and K.M. Hilliard. "Depression and Anxiety among Asian American Elders: A Review of the Literature." *Clinical Psychology Review* 19, no. 3 (1999): 343–57.

46. Okazaki, S. "Sources of Ethnic Differences between Asian American and White American College Students on Measures of Depression and Social Anxiety." *Journal of Abnormal Psychology* 106, no. 1 (1997): 52–60.

47. Lau, A.S., J. Fung, S. Wang, and S. Kang. "Explaining Elevated Social Anxiety among Asian Americans: Emotional Attunement and a Cultural Double Bind." *Cultural Diversity and Ethnic Minority Psychology* 15, no. 1 (2009): 77–85.

48. Li, S. Tinsley, T. Edwards, S. Dhaliwas, J. Armstrong, and J.Y. Ao. "Anxiety and Depression in Asian Americans: Stress and Cultural Values." Paper presented at the Midwestern Psychological Association Convention. Chicago, Illinois, 2006.

49. Hilliard, K.M., and G.Y. Iwamasa. "The Conceptualization of Anxiety: An Exploratory Study of Japanese Older Adults." *Journal of Clinical Gerontology* 7, no. 1 (2001): 53–65.

50. Singh, M., S. Arteaga, and M.C. Zea. "Factors Related to Depression and Anxiety among East and South Asian American Women." Paper presented at conference Enhancing Outcomes in Women's Health: Translating Psychosocial Behavioral Research into Primary Care. Washington, DC: American Psychological Association, 2002.

51. Hwang, W.-C., and S. Goto. "The Impact of Perceived Racial Discrimination on the Mental Health of Asian American and Latino College Students." *Cultural Diversity and Ethnic Minority Psychology* 14, no. 4 (2008): 326–35.

52. Febles, F., and S. Milan. "Unraveling the Latino Paradox: Psychiatric Risk Depends on Regional Origins." Paper presented at the American Psychological Association Annual Convention, Boston, Massachusetts, August 14–17, 2008.

53. Weinrich, J. D. Jr., J. H. Atkinson, J. A. McCutchan, and I. Grant. "Is Gender Dysphoria Dysphoric? Elevated Depression and Anxiety in Gender Dysphoric and Nondysphoric Homosexual and Bisexual Men in an HIV Sample." *Archives of Sexual Behavior* 24 (1995): 55–72.

54. Martell, C. R., M. Botzer, M. Williams, and D. Yashimoto. "Gay, Lesbian, Transgender and Bisexual Individuals." Working Paper, University of Washington, 2009.

55. Pachankis, John E., and Marvin R. Goldfried. "Social Anxiety in Young Gay Men." *Journal of Anxiety Disorders* 20, no. 8 (2006): 996–1015.

56. Rosmarin, David H., Elizabeth J. Krumrei, and Gerhard Anderson. "Religion as a Predictor of Psychological Distress in Two Religious Communities." *Cognitive Behavior Therapy* 38, no. 1 (2009): 54–64.

CHAPTER 4

1. Crowe, R. R. Jr., R. Noyes, D. L. Pauls, and D. Slyman. "A Family Study of Panic Disorder." *Archives of General Psychiatry* 40 (1983): 1065–69.

2. Beidel, D. C., and S. M. Turner. *Childhood Anxiety Disorders: A Guide to Research and Treatment.* New York: Routledge, 2005.

3. Fyer, A. J., S. Mannuzza, M. S. Gallops, L. Y. Martin, C. Aaronson, J. M. Gorman, M. R. Liebowitz, and D. F. Klein. "Familial Transmission of Simple Phobias and Fears." *Archives of General Psychiatry* 47 (1990): 252–56.

4. Torgersen, S. "Genetic Factors in Anxiety Disorders." *Archives of General Psychiatry* 40, no. 10 (1983): 1085–89.

5. Hettema, J. M., C. A. Prescott, J. M. Myers, M. C. Neale, and K. S. Kendler. "The Structure of Genetic and Environmental Risk Factors for Anxiety Disorders in Men and Women." *Archives of General Psychiatry* 62 (2005): 182–89.

6. Leckman, J. F., and Y.-S. Kim. "A Primary Candidate Gene for Obsessive-Compulsive Disorder." *Archives of General Psychiatry* 63 (2006): 717–20.

7. Denys, D., F. Van Nieuwerburgh, D. Deforce, and H.G.M. Westenberg. "Prediction of Response to Paroxetine and Venlafaxine by Serotonin-Related Genes in Obsessive-Compulsive Disorder in Randomized, Double-Blind Trial." *Journal of Clinical Psychiatry* 68 (2007): 747–53.

8. Eysenck, H. J., ed. *The Biological Basis of Personality.* Springfield, IL: Charles C. Thomas, 1967.

9. Kendler, K. S., R. C. Kessler, E. E. Walters, C. MacLean, M. C. Neale, A. C. Heath, and L. J. Eaves. "Stressful Life Events, Genetic Liability, and Onset of an Episode of Major Depression in Women." *American Journal of Psychiatry* 152 (1995): 833–42.

10. Barlow, D. H. *Anxiety and Its Disorders: The Nature and Treatment of Anxiety and Panic.* 2nd ed. New York: Guilford Press, 2002.

11. Craske, M. G., and D. H. Barlow. "Panic Disorder and Agoraphobia." In *Clinical Handbook of Psychological Disorders*, edited by David H. Barlow, 1–47. New York: Guilford Press, 1993.

12. Goddard, A. W., and D. S. Charney. "Toward an Integrated Neurobiology of Panic Disorder." *Journal of Clinical Psychiatry* 58, Suppl. 2 (1997): 4–12.

13. Damsa, C., M. Kosel, and J. Moussally. "Current Status of Brain Imaging in Anxiety Disorders." *Current Opinion in Psychiatry* 22, no. 1 (2009): 96–110.

14. Charney, D. S., and W. C. Drevetts. "Neurobiological Basis of Anxiety Disorders." In *Neuropsychopharmocology: The Fifth Generation of Progress*, edited by K. L. Davis, D. Charney, J. T. Coyle, and C. Nemeroff, 901–51. Philadelphia: Lippincott, Williams & Wilkins, 2002.

15. Gray, J. A. "Issues in the Neuropsychology of Anxiety." In *Anxiety and the Anxiety Disorders*, edited by A. H. Tuma and J. D. Maser. Hillsdale, NJ: Erlbaum, 1985.

16. Gray, J. A., and N. McNaughton. "The Neuropsychology of Anxiety: Reprise." In *Perspectives on Anxiety, Panic and Fear*, edited by D. A. Hope, 61–134. Lincoln: University of Nebraska Press, 1996.

17. McNally, R. J. *Panic Disorder: A Critical Analysis*. New York: Guilford Press, 1994.

18. Tancer, M. E., R. B. Mailman, M. B. Stein, G. A. Mason, S. W. Carson, and R. N. Golden. "Neuroendocrine Responsivity to Monaminergic System Probes in Generalized Social Phobia." *Anxiety* 1, no. 5 (1994): 216–23.

19. Schweizer, E., K. Rickels, S. Weiss, and S. Zavodnick. "Maintenance Drug Treatment of Panic Disorder: I. Results of a Prospective, Placebo-Controlled Comparison of Alprazolam and Imipramine." *Archives of General Psychiatry* 50, no. 1 (1993): 51–60.

20. Kim, Y-K., H-J. Lee, J-C. Yang, J-A. Hwang, and H-K. Yoon. "A Tryptophan Hydoxylase 2 Gene Polymorphism Is Associated with Panic Disorder." *Behavior Genetics* 39, no. 2 (2009): 170–75.

21. Francis, D. D., J. Diorio, P. M. Plotsky, and M. J. Meaney. "Environmental Enrichment Reverses the Effects of Maternal Separation on Stress Reactivity." *Journal of Neuroscience* 22, no. 18 (2002): 7840–43.

22. Johnson, B. A., J. D. Roache, M. A. Javors, C. C. DiClemente, C. R. Cloninger, T. J. Prihoda, P. S. Bordnick, N. Ait-Daoud, and J. Hensler. "Ondansetron for Reduction of Drinking among Biologically Predisposed Alcoholic Patients." *Journal of the American Medical Association* 284, no. 8 (2000): 963–71.

23. Koffel, E., and D. Watson. "The Two-Factor Structure of Sleep Complaints and Its Relations to Depression and Anxiety." *Journal of Abnormal Psychology* 118, no. 1 (2009): 183–94.

24. Freud, S. *New Introductory Lectures in Psychoanalysis*. Edited by James Strachey, *The Complete Works of Sigmund Freud*. New York: W. W. Norton, 1965.

25. Chorpita, B. F., and D. H. Barlow. "The Development of Anxiety: The Role of Control in the Early Environment." *Psychological Bulletin* 124, no. 1 (1998): 3–21.

26. Rogers, C. R. *On Becoming a Person*. New York: Houghton Mifflin, 1961.

27. Watson, J. B., and R. Rayner. "Conditional Emotional Reactions." *Journal of Experimental Psychology* 3 (1920): 1–14.

28. Rachman, S. "The Conditioning Theory of Fear-Acquisition: A Critical Examination." *Behavior Research and Therapy* 15 (1977): 583–89.

29. Mowrer, O.H. "Stimulus Response Theory of Anxiety." *Psychological Review* 46 (1939): 553–65.

30. Rachman, S. *Fear and Courage.* 2nd ed. New York: Freeman, 1990.

31. Bandura, A. *Principles of Behavior Modification.* New York: Holt, Rinehart, & Winston, 1969.

32. Agras, W.S., D. Sylvester, and D. Oliveau. "The Epidemiology of Common Fears and Phobias." *Comprehensive Psychiatry* 10 (1969): 151–56.

33. Poulton, R., and R.G. Menzies. "Non-Associative Fear Acquisition: A Review of the Evidence from Retrospective and Longitudinal Research." *Behavior Research and Therapy* 40 (2002): 127–49.

34. Seligman, M. "Phobias and Preparedness." *Behavior Therapy* 2 (1971): 307–20.

35. Kagan, J., J.S. Reznick, C. Clarke, N. Snidman, and C. Garcia-Coll. "Behavioral Inhibition to the Unfamiliar." *Child Development* 55 (1984): 2212–25.

36. Bruch, M.A., and R.G. Heimberg. "Differences in Perceptions of Parental and Personal Characteristics between Generalized and Nongeneralized Social Phobics." *Journal of Anxiety Disorders* 8 (1994): 155–68.

37. Antony, M. M, C.L. Purdon, V. Huta, and R.P. Swinson. "Dimensions of Perfectionism across the Anxiety Disorders." *Behavior Research and Therapy* 36 (1998): 1143–54.

38. Fransella, F., ed. *An International Handbook of Personal Construct Psychology.* New York: John Wiley, 2003.

39. Ellis, A. *Reason and Emotion in Psychotherapy.* Secaucus, NJ: Prentice-Hall, 1962.

40. Beck, A.T., and G. Emery. *Anxiety Disorders and Phobias: A Cognitive Perspective.* New York: Basic Books, 1985.

41. Goldstein, A.J., and D.L. Chambless. "A Reanalysis of Agoraphobia." *Behavior Therapy* 9 (1978): 47–59.

42. Reiss, S., and R.J. McNally. "The Expectancy Model of Fear." In *Theoretical Issues in Behavior Therapy,* edited by S. Reiss and R.R. Bootzin, 107–21. New York: Academic Press, 1985.

43. Koster, E.H. W., E. Fox, and C. MacLeod. "Introduction to the Special Section on Cognitive Bias Modification in Emotional Disorders." *Journal of Abnormal Psychology* 118, no. 1 (2009): 1–4.

44. McNally, R.F., and H. Reese. "Information-Processing Approaches to Understanding Anxiety Disorders." In *Handbook of Anxiety and Related Disorders,* edited by Martin M. Antony and Murray B. Stein, 136–52. New York: Oxford University Press, 2009.

45. Schmidt, Norman B., Richey J. Anthony, Julia D. Buckner, and Kiara R. Timpano. "Attention Training for Generalized Social Anxiety Disorder." *Journal of Abnormal Psychology* 118, no. 1 (2009): 5–14.

46. Kindt, M., and J.F. Brosschot. "Cognitive Bias in Spider-Phobic Children: Comparison of a Pictorial and a Linguistic Spider Stoop." *Journal of Psychopathology and Behavioral Assessment* 21 (1999): 207–20.

47. Yartz, A.R., and M.J. Zvolensky. "Panic-Relevant Predictability Preferences: A Laboratory Task." *Journal of Abnormal Psychology* 117 (2008): 242–46.

48. Beaudreau, S.A., and R. O'Hara. "The Association of Anxiety and Depressive Symptoms with Cognitive Performance in Community-Dwelling Older Adults." *Psychology and Aging* 24, no. 2 (2009): 507–12.

49. Gorman, J., J.M. Kent, G.M. Sullivan, and J.D. Coplan. "Neuroanatomical Hypothesis of Panic Disorder, Revised." *American Journal of Psychiatry* 157 (2000): 493–505.

50. Lonsdorf, T.B., and A.I. Weike. "Genetic Gating of Human Fear Learning and Extinction: Possible Implications for Gene-Environment Interaction in Anxiety Disorder." *Psychological Science* 20, no. 2 (2009): 198–206.

51. Bouton, M.E., S. Mineka, and D.H. Barlow. "A Modern Learning Theory Perspective on the Etiology of Panic Disorder." *Psychological Review* 108 (2001): 4–32.

52. Suomi, S.J. "Anxiety in Young Nonhuman Primates." In *Anxiety Disorders of Childhood*, edited by R. Gittelman, 1–23. New York: Guilford Press, 1986.

53. Kagan, J., J.S. Reznick, and N. Snidman. "Biological Bases of Childhood Shyness." *Science* 240 (1988): 167–71.

54. Turner, S.M., D.C. Beidel, J.W. Borden, M.A. Stanley, and R.G. Jacob. "Social Phobia: Axis I and II Correlates." *Journal of Abnormal Psychology* 100 (1991): 102–6.

55. Crowe, R.R., D.L. Pauls, D.J. Slymen, and R. Noyes. "A Family Study of Anxiety Neurosis." *Archives of General Psychiatry* 37 (1980): 77–79.

56. Huffman, Jeff C., Felicia A. Smith, Mark A. Blais, James L. Januzzi, and Gregory L. Fricchione. "Anxiety, Independent of Depressive Symptoms, Is Associated with In-Hospital Cardiac Complications after Acute Myocardial Infarction." *Journal of Psychosomatic Research* 65, no. 6 (2008): 557–63.

57. Chorney, D.B., M.F. Detweiler, and T.L. Morris. "The Interplay of Sleep Disturbance, Anxiety, and Depression in Children." *Journal of Pediatric Psychology* 33 (2008): 339–48.

58. Milrod, B.L., F.N. Busch, A.M. Cooper, and T. Shapiro. *Manual of Panic-Focused Psychodynamic Psychotherapy*. Washington, DC: American Psychiatric Association, 1997.

59. Schafer, I., C.A. Ross, and J. Read. "Childhood Trauma in Psychotic and Dissociative Disorders." In *Psychosis, Trauma, and Dissociation: Emerging Perspectives on Severe Psychopathology*, edited by Andrew Moskowitz, Ingo Schafer, and Martin J. Dorahy, 137–50. New York: Wiley-Blackwell, 2008.

60. Cabizuca, M., C. Marques-Portella, M.V. Mendlowicz, E.S.G. Coutinho, and I. Firueira. "Posttraumatic Stress Disorder in Parents of Children with Chronic Illness: A Meta-Analysis." *Health Psychology* 25, no. 3 (2009): 379–88.

CHAPTER 5

1. University of Maryland Medical Center. "Anxiety Disorders." *Medical References; Patient Education* (2008), http://www.umn.edu/patiented/articles/what_anxiety_disorders_000028-1.htm.

2. Psychiatry.HealthSE.com. "Generalized Anxiety Disorder (GAD)." *Current Medical Diagnosis & Treatment in Psychiatry* (2005), http://psychiatry.healthse.com/psy/more/generalised_anxiety_disorder_gad/.

3. Wittchen, H.U., V. Reed, and R.C. Kessler. "The Relationship of Agoraphobia and Panic in a Community Sample of Adolescents and Young Adults." *Archives of General Psychiatry* 55 (1998): 1017–24.

4. Swartz, Karen I. "Depression and Anxiety." In *The Johns Hopkins White Papers*. Baltimore: Johns Hopkins Medical School, 2007.

5. American Psychiatric Association. *Diagnostic and Statistical Manual, Fourth Edition, Text Revision*. Washington, DC: American Psychiatric Association, 2000.

6. Rapee, R.M. "Generalized Anxiety Disorder: A Review of Clinical Features and Theoretical Concepts." *Clinical Psychology Review* 11 (1991): 419–40.

7. Sanderson, W.C., and D.H. Barlow. "A Description of Patients Diagnosed with DSM-III-R Generalized Anxiety Disorder." *Journal of Nervous and Mental Disorders* 178 (1990): 588–91.

8. American Psychiatric Association. *Diagnostic and Statistical Manual, Third Edition, Revised*. Washington, DC: American Psychiatric Association, 1994.

9. Bernstein, G.A., and C.M. Borchardt. "Anxiety Disorders of Childhood and Adolescence: A Critical Review." *Journal of the American Academy of Child and Adolescent Psychiatry* 30, no. 4 (1991): 519–32.

10. Brawman-Mintzer, O., and R.B. Lydiard. "Psychopharmacology of Anxiety Disorders." *Psychiatric Clinics of North America* 1 (1994): 51–79.

11. Tollefson, G.D., M.G. Luxenberg, R. Valentine, G. Dunsmore, and S.L. Tollefson. "An Open Label Trial of Alprazolam in Comorbid Irritable Bowel Syndrome and Generalized Anxiety Disorder." *Journal of Clinical Psychiatry* 52, no. 12 (1991): 502–8.

12. Carter, C.S., and R.J. Maddock. "Chest Pain in Generalized Anxiety Disorder." *International Journal of Psychiatry in Medicine* 22, no. 3 (1992): 291–98.

13. Kushner, M.G. "Relationship between Alcohol Problems and Anxiety Disorders." *American Journal of Psychiatry* 153, no. 1 (1996): 139.

14. Fisher, Peter L., and Adrian Wells. "Psychological Models of Worry and Generalized Anxiety Disorder." In *Oxford Handbook of Anxiety and Related Disorders*, edited by Martin M. Antony and Murray B. Stein, 225–37. New York: Oxford University Press, 2009.

15. Hazlett-Stevens, Holly, Larry D. Pruitt, and Angela Collins. "Phenomenology of Generalized Anxiety Disorder." In *Oxford Handbook of Anxiety and Related Disorders*, edited by Martin M. Antony and Murray B. Stein, 47–55. New York: Oxford University Press, 2009.

16. Pluess, M., C. Ansgar, and F.H. Wilhelm. "Muscle Tension in Generalized Anxiety Disorder: A Critical Review of the Literature." *Journal of Anxiety Disorders* 23, no. 1 (2009): 1–11.

17. Robichaud, M., and M.J. Dugas. "Psychological Treatment of Generalized Anxiety Disorder." In *Oxford Handbook of Anxiety and Related Disorders*, edited by Martin M. Antony and Murray B. Stein, 364–74. New York: Oxford University Press, 2009.

18. Amir, N., C. Beard, M. Burns, and J. Bomyea. "Attention Modification Program in Individuals with Generalized Anxiety Disorder." *Journal of Abnormal Psychology* 118, no. 1 (2009): 28–33.

19. Markowitz, J.S., M.M. Weissman, R. Oullette, J.D. Lish, and G. Klerman. "Quality of Life in Panic Disorder." *Archives of General Psychiatry* 46 (1989): 984–82.

20. Clark, D.M. "A Cognitive Approach to Panic." *Behavioral Research and Therapy* 24, (1986): 461–70.

21. Norton, P. J. "Integrated Psychological Treatment of Multiple Anxiety Disorders." In *Oxford Handbook of Anxiety and Related Disorders*, edited by Martin M. Antony and Murray B. Stein. New York: Oxford University Press, 2009.

22. Brown, T. A., and E. A. Deagle. "Structured Interview Assessment of Nonclinical Panic." *Behavior Therapy* 23 (1992): 75–85.

23. Oei, T.P.S., K. Wanstall, and L. Evans. "Sex Differences in Panic Disorder and Agoraphobia." *Journal of Anxiety Disorders* 4 (1990): 317–24.

24. First, M. B., and A. Tasman. "Anxiety Disorders: Social and Specific Phobias." In *DSM-IV-TR Mental Disorders: Diagnosis, Etiology, and Treatment*, edited by M. B. First and A. Tasman, 867–901. Chichester, England: John Wiley, 2004.

25. Reiss, S., and R. J. McNally. "The Expectancy Model of Fear." In *Theoretical Issues in Behavior Therapy*, edited by S. Reiss and R. R. Bootzin, 107–21. New York: Academic Press, 1985.

26. Rouillon, F. "Epidemiology of Panic Disorder." *Human Psychopharmacology* 12 (1997): S7–S12.

27. Eaton, W. W., R. C. Kessler, H. U. Wittchen, and W. J. Magee. "Panic and Panic Disorder in the United States." *American Journal of Psychiatry* 151 (1994): 413–20.

28. Weissman, Myrna M., Roger C. Bland, Glorisa J. Canino, Carlo Faravelli, Steven Greenwald, Hai-Gwo Hwu, Peter R. Joyce, Elie G. Karam, Chung-Kyoon Lee, Joseph Lellouch, Jean-Pierre Lépine, Stephen C. Newman, Mark A. Oakley-Browne, Maritza Rubio-Stipec, J. Elisabeth Wells, Priya J. Wickramaratne, Hans-Ulrich Wittchen, and Eng-Kung Yeh. "The Cross-National Epidemiology of Panic Disorder." *Archives of General Psychiatry* 54, no. 4 (1997): 305–9.

29. Ballenger, J. C., and A. J. Fryer. "Panic Disorder and Agoraphobia." In *DSM-IV Sourcebook*, edited by T. A. Widiger, A. J. Frances, H. A. Pincus, R. Ross, M. B. First, and W. W. Davis, 411–71. Washington, DC: American Psychiatric Association, 1996.

30. McCabe, L., J. Cairney, S. Veldhuizen, N. Herrmann, and D.L. Streiner. "Prevalence and Correlates of Agoraphobia in Older Adults." *American Journal of Geriatric Psychiatry* 14, no. 6 (2006): 515.

31. National Institute of Mental Health. *Anxiety Disorders*. Washington, DC: National Institute of Mental Health, 2009.

32. Keller, M. B., K. A. Yonkers, M. G. Warshaw, J. Gollan, A. O. Massion, K. White, A. Swartz, L. Pratt, J. Reich, and P. W. Larori. "Remission and Relapse in Subjects with Panic Disorder and Panic with Agoraphobia." *Journal of Nervous and Mental Disorders* 182 (1991): 290–96.

33. Chen, J., M. Tschiya, N. Kawakami, and T. A. Funukawa. "Non-Fearful vs. Fearful Panic Attacks: A General Population Study from the National Comorbidity Survey." *Journal of Affective Disorders* 112, no. 1–3 (2009): 273–78.

34. Psychiatry.HealthSE.com. "Panic Disorder and Agoraphobia." *Current Medical Diagnosis and Treatment in Psychiatry* (2005), http://psychiatry.healthse.com/psy/more/panic_disorder_and_agoraphobia/.

35. Weissman, M. M. "Panic Disorder: Impact on Quality of Life." *Journal of Clinical Psychiatry* 52 (1991): 6–9.

36. Katerndahl, D. A., and J. P. Realini. "Where Do Panic Attack Sufferers Seek Care?" *Journal of Family Practice* 40 (1995): 237–43.

37. Boyd, J.H. "Use of Mental Health Services for the Treatment of Panic Disorder." *American Journal of Psychiatry* 143 (1986): 1569–74.

38. Greenberg, P.E., T. Sisitsky, R.C. Kessler, S.N. Finkelstein, E.R. Berndt, J.R.T. Davidson, J.C. Ballenger, and A.J. Fyer. "The Economic Burden of Anxiety Disorders in the 1990's." *Journal of Clinical Psychiatry* 60, no. 7 (1999): 427–35.

39. Ohtani, T., H. Kaiya, T. Utsumi, K. Inoue, N. Kato, and T. Sasaki. "Sensitivity to Seasonal Changes in Panic Disorder Patients." *Psychiatry and Clinical Neurosciences* 60 (2006): 379–83.

40. Teng, E.J., A.D. Chaison, S.D. Bailey, J.D. Hamilton, and N.J. Dunn. "When Anxiety Symptoms Masquerade as Medical Symptoms: What Medical Specialists Know about Panic Disorder and Available Psychological Treatments." *Journal of Clinical Psychology in Medical Settings* 15, no. 4 (2008): 314–21.

41. Busch, F.N., B.L. Milrod, and L.S. Sandberg. "A Study Demonstrating Efficacy of a Psychoanalytic Psychotherapy for Panic Disorder: Implications for Psychoanalytic Research, Theory, and Practice." *Journal of the American Psychoanalytic Association* 57, no. 1 (2009): 131–48.

CHAPTER 6

1. Davey, G.C.L., and S. Marzillier. "Disgust and Animal Phobias." In *Disgust and Its Disorders: Theory, Assessment, and Treatment Implications*, edited by B.O. Olatunje and D. McKay, 169–90. Washington, DC: American Psychological Association, 2009.

2. First, M.B., and A. Tasman. "Anxiety Disorders: Social and Specific Phobias." In *DSM-IV-TR Mental Disorders: Diagnosis, Etiology, and Treatment*, edited by M.B. First and A. Tasman, 867–901. Chichester, England: John Wiley, 2004.

3. Eaton, W.W., A. Dryman, and M.M. Weissman. "Panic and Phobia: The Diagnosis of Panic Disorder." In *Psychiatric Disorders in America: The Epidemiologic Catchment Area Study*, edited by L.N. Robins and D.A. Reiger, 155–79. New York: Free Press, 1991.

4. National Institute of Mental Health. *Anxiety Disorders*. Washington, DC: National Institute of Mental Health, 2009.

5. Psychiatry.HealthSE.com. "Specific Phobias." *Current Medical Diagnosis & Treatment in Psychiatry* (2005), http://psychiatry.healthse.com/psy/more/specific_phobias/.

6. Curtis, G.C., W.J. McGee, W.W. Eaton, H.U. Wittchen, and R.C. Kessler. "Specific Fears and Phobias: Epidemiology and Classification." *British Journal of Psychiatry* 173 (1998): 212–17.

7. Ost, L-G. "Blood and Injection Phobia: Background and Cognitive, Physiological, and Behavioral Variables." *Journal of Abnormal Psychology* 101 (1992): 68–74.

8. Psychiatry.HealthSE.com. "Social Phobias." *Current Medical Diagnosis & Treatment in Psychiatry* (2005), http://psychiatry.healthse.com/psy/more/social_phobia.

9. Swartz, K. "Depression and Anxiety." In *The Johns Hopkins White Papers*. Baltimore: Johns Hopkins Medical School, 2007.

10. Antony, M.M., and R.P. Swinson. *Phobic Disorders and Panic in Adults: A Guide to Assessment and Treatment*. Washington, DC: American Psychological Association, 2000.

11. Turk, C.L., R.G. Heimberg, S.M. Orsillo, C.S. Holt, A. Gitow, L.L. Street, F.R. Schneier, and M.R. Liebowitz. "An Investigation of Gender Differences in Social Phobia." *Journal of Anxiety Disorders* 12 (1998): 209–23.

12. "Social Phobia." *Harvard Mental Health Letter*. Boston: Harvard Medical School, 1994.

13. Heiser, N.A., S.M. Turner, D.C. Beidel, and R. Roberson-Nay. "Differentiating Social Phobia from Shyness." *Journal of Anxiety Disorders* 23, no. 4 (2009): 469–76.

14. Turner, S.M., D.C. Beidel, and R.M. Townsley. "Social Phobia: A Comparison of Specific and Generalized Subtype and Avoidant Personality Disorder." *Journal of Abnormal Psychology* 101, no. 2 (1992): 326–31.

15. "Rethinking Posttraumatic Stress Disorder." *Harvard Mental Health Letter*. Boston: Harvard Medical School, 2007.

16. Kessler, R.C., A. Sonnega, E. Bromet, M. Hughes, and C.B. Nelson. "Posttraumatic Stress Disorder in the National Comorbidity Survey." *Archives of General Psychiatry* 52 (1995): 1048–60.

17. Breslau, N. "The Epidemiology of Posttraumatic Stress Disorder: What Is the Extent of the Problem?" *Journal of Clinical Psychiatry* 62 (2001): 16–22.

18. American Psychiatric Association. *Diagnostic and Statistical Manual, Fourth Edition, Text Revision*. Washington, DC: American Psychiatric Association, 2000.

19. Weiss, D.S. "Posttraumatic Stress Disorder: Part 1." In *PTSD: In an Age of Violence, Terror, and Disaster*, 1–3. Audio CD. San Francisco: Audio-Digest Psychiatry, 2008.

20. Norris, F.H. "Epidemiology of Trauma: Frequency and Impact of Different Potentially Traumatic Events on Different Demographic Events." *Journal of Consulting and Clinical Psychology* 60 (1992): 409–18.

21. March, J.S. "The Nosology of Posttraumatic Stress Disorder." *Journal of Anxiety Disorders* 4 (1990): 61–82.

22. Shalev, A., A. Bleich, and R.J. Ursano. "Posttraumatic Stress Disorder: Somatic Comorbidity and Effort Tolerance." *Psychosomatics* 31 (1990): 197–303.

23. Nydegger, R.V., L.A. Nydegger, and F. Basile. "Posttraumatic Stress Disorder and Coping in Career Professional Firefighters." Paper presented at the International Business and Economic Research Conference, Las Vegas, Nevada, October 2010.

24. Psychiatry.HealthSE.com. "Post-Traumatic Stress Disorder (PTSD)." *Current Medical Diagnosis and Treatment in Psychiatry* (2005), http://psychiatry.healthse.com/psy/more/post_traumatic_stress_disorder_ptsd/.

25. Schnurr, P.P., and M.K. Jankowski. "Physical Health and Posttraumatic Stress Disorder: Review and Synthesis." *Seminars in Clinical Neuropsychiatry* 4 (1999): 295–304.

26. University of Maryland Medical Center. "Anxiety Disorders." *Medical References; Patient Education* (2008), http://www.umn.edu/patiented/articles/what_anxiety_disorders_000028---1.htm.

27. Harvey, A.G., and R.A. Bryant. "Dissociative Symptoms in Acute Stress Disorder." *Journal of Traumatic Stress* 12, no. 4 (1999): 573–680.

28. Koopman, C., C. Classen, and D. Spiegel. "Predictors of Posttraumatic Stress Symptoms among Survivors of the Oakland/Berkeley, California Firestorm." *American Journal of Psychiatry* 151 (1994): 888–94.

29. Marshall, R. D., R. Spitzer, and M. R. Liebowitz. "Review and Critique of the New DSM-IV Diagnosis of Acute Stress Disorder." *American Journal of Psychiatry* 156 (1999): 1677–88.

30. Elwood, L. S., K. S. Hahn, B. O. Olatunji, and N. L. Williams. "Cognitive Vulnerabilities to the Development of PTSD: A Review of Four Vulnerabilities and the Proposal of an Integrative Vulnerability Model." *Clinical Psychology Review* 29, no. 1 (2009): 87–100.

31. Pitman, R. K. "Biological Findings in Posttraumatic Stress Disorder: Implications for DSM-IV Classification." In *Posttraumatic Stress Disorder: DSM-IV and Beyond*, edited by E. B. Foa, 173–90. Washington, DC: American Psychiatric Press, 1993.

32. Rauch, S. L., P. J. Whalen, L. M. Shin, S. C. McInerney, M. L. Macklin, N. B. Lasko, S. P. Orr, and R. K. Pitman. "Exaggerated Amygdala Response to Masked Facial Stimuli in Posttraumatic Stress Disorder: A Functional MRI Study." *Biological Psychiatry* 47 (2000): 769–76.

33. Lieberzon, I., S. F. Taylor, R. Amdur, T. D. Jung, K. R. Chamberlain, S. Minoshima, R. A. Koeppe, and L. M. Fig. "Brain Activation in PTSD in Response to Trauma-Related Stimuli." *Biological Psychiatry* 45 (1999): 817–26.

34. Shin, L. M., R. J. McNally, S. M. Kosslin, W. L. Thompson, S. L. Rauch, N. M. Alpert, L. J. Metzger, N. B. Lasko, S. P. Orr, and R. K. Pitman. "Regional Cerebral Blood Flow during Script-Driven Imagery in Childhood Sexual Abuse-Related PTSD: A Pet Investigation." *American Journal of Psychiatry* 156 (1999): 575–84.

35. Yehuda, R., E. L. Giller, S. M. Southwick, and J. W. Mason. "Hypothalamic-Pituitary-Adrenal Dysfunction in Posttraumatic Stress Disorder." *Biological Psychiatry* 44 (1991): 266–74.

36. Solomon, S. D., E. T. Gerrity, and A. M. Muff. "Efficacy of Treatments for Posttraumatic Stress Disorder: An Empirical Review." *Journal of the American Medical Association* 268 (1992): 633–38.

37. Davidson, J. R., L. A. Tupler, W. H. Wilson, and K. M. Connor. "A Family Study of Chronic Posttraumatic Stress Disorder Following Rape Trauma." *Journal of Psychiatric Research* 32 (1998): 301–9.

38. Hidalgo, R. B., and J.R.T. Davidson. "Selective Serotonin-Reuptake Inhibitors in Post-Traumatic Stress Disorder." *Journal of Psychopharmacology* 14, no. 1 (2000): 70–76.

39. Riggs, D. S., and E. B. Foa. "Psychological Treatment of Posttraumatic Stress Disorder and Acute Stress Disorder." In *Oxford Handbook of Anxiety and Related Disorders*, edited by Martin M. Antony and Murray B. Stein, 417–28. New York: Oxford University Press, 2009.

40. Lundin, T. "The Treatment of Acute Trauma: Posttraumatic Stress Disorder Prevention." *Psychiatric Clinics of North America* 17 (1994): 385–91.

41. Warda, G., and R. A. Bryant. "Thought Control Strategies in Acute Stress Disorder." *Behavior Research and Therapy* 36 (1998): 1171–75.

42. Miller, Michael Craig. "Preventing PTSD." *Harvard Mental Health Letter*. Boston: Harvard Mental Health Letter, 2009.

43. Monson, Candice M. "Conjoint Treatment for PTSD." In *Second Annual Posttraumatic Stress Disorder Symposium*, 2–3. Audio CD. Cleveland, OH: Audio-Digest Psychiatry, 2007.

44. Rasmussen, S.A., and J.L. Eisen. "Phenomenology of Obsessive-Compulsive Disorder." In *Psychology of Obsessive-Compulsive Disorder*, edited by J. Insel and S. Rasmussen, 743–58. New York: Springer-Verlag, 1991.

45. Swedo, S.E., J.L. Rapoport, J. Leonard, M. Lenane, and D. Cheslow. "Obsessive-Compulsive Disorder in Children and Adolescents: Clinical Phenomenology of 70 Consecutive Cases." *Archives of General Psychiatry* 46 (1989): 335–41.

46. Leonard, H.I., M.C. Lenane, S.E. Swedo, D.C. Rettew, E.S. Gershon, and J.L. Rapoport. "Tics and Tourette's Disorder: A 2- to 7-Year Follow-up of 54 Obsessive-Compulsive Children." *American Journal of Psychiatry* 149, no. 9 (1992): 1244–51.

47. Robertson, M.M., M.R. Trimble, and A.J. Lees. "The Psychopathology of the Gilles De La Tourette's Syndrome: A Phenomenological Analysis." *British Journal of Psychology* 152 (1988): 283–90.

48. Eisen, J.L., D.A. Beer, M.T. Pato, T.A. Venditto, and S.A. Rasmussen. "Obsessive-Compulsive Disorder in Schizophrenia and Schizoaffective Disorders." *American Journal of Psychiatry* 154, no. 2 (1997): 271–73.

49. Myers, J.K., M.M Weissman, G.L. Tischler, C.E. Holzer III, P.J. Lear, J. Orvaschel, J.C. Anthony, J.H. Boyd Jr., J.D. Burke, M. Kramer, and R. Stoltzman. "Six-Month Prevalence of Psychiatric Disorders in Three Communities, 1980 to 1982." *Archives of General Psychiatry* 41 (1984): 959–67.

50. Nestadt, G., J. Samuels, M. Riddle, O.J. Bienvenu III, K-Y. Liang, M. LaBuda, J. Walkup, M. Grados, and R. Hoen-Saric. "A Family Study of Obsessive-Compulsive Disorder." *Archives of General Psychiatry* 57 (2000): 358–63.

51. Saxena, L., A.L. Brody, J.M. Schwartz, and L.R. Baxter. "Neuroimaging and Front-Subcortical Circuitry in Obsessive-Compulsive Disorder." *British Journal of Psychiatry* 173, Suppl. 35 (1998): 26–37.

52. Pigott, T.A. "OCD: Where the Serotonin Selective Story Begins." *Journal of Clinical Psychiatry* 57, Suppl. 6 (1996): 11–20.

53. Griest, J.H., J.W. Jefferson, K.A. Koback, D.J. Katzelnick, and R.C. Serlin. "Efficacy and Tolerability of Serotonin Transport Inhibitors in Obsessive-Compulsive Disorder." *Archives of General Psychiatry* 52 (1998): 53–60.

54. Rasmussen, S.A., and M.T. Tsuang. "Clinical Characteristics and Family History in DSM-III Obsessive-Compulsive Disorder." *American Journal of Psychiatry* 143 (1986): 317–22.

55. Pauls, D.L., J.P. Alsobrook, W. Goodman, S. Rasmussen, and J.F. Leckman. "A Family Study of Obsessive-Compulsive Disorder." *American Journal of Psychiatry* 152 (1995): 76–84.

56. Pauls, D.L., K.E. Towbin, J.F. Leckman, G.E.P. Zahner, and D.J. Cohen. "Gilles de la Tourette's Syndrome and Obsessive-Compulsive Disorder: Evidence Supporting a Genetic Relationship." *Archives of General Psychiatry* 43 (1986): 1180–82.

57. Pauls, D.L. "Phenotypic Variability in Obsessive-Compulsive Disorder and Its Relationship to Familial Risk." *CNS Spectrums* 4, no. 6 (1999): 32–48.

58. Baer, L., and W.E. Minichiello. "Behavior Therapy for Obsessive-Compulsive Disorder." In *Obsessive-Compulsive Disorders: Theory and Management*, edited by M.A. Jenike, L. Baer and W.E. Minichiello. St. Louis: Year Book Medical Publishers, 1990.

59. Cohen, I.J., and I. Galykner. "Towards an Integration of Psychological and Biological Models of Obsessive-Compulsive Disorder: Phylogenetics Considerations." *CNS Spectrums* 2, no. 10 (1997): 26–44.

CHAPTER 7

1. Chavira, D. A., M. B. Stein, and P. Roy-Hyrne. "Managing Anxiety in Primary Care." In *Oxford Handbook of Anxiety and Related Disorders*, edited by Martin M. Antony and Murray B. Stein, 512–22. New York: Oxford University Press, 2009.

2. Kushner, M. G. "Relationship between Alcohol Problems and Anxiety Disorders." *American Journal of Psychiatry* 153, no. 1 (1996): 139.

3. Swartz, K. "Depression and Anxiety." In *The Johns Hopkins White Papers*. Baltimore: Johns Hopkins Medical School, 2007.

4. Otto, M. W., E. Behar, J.A.J. Smits, and S. G. Hoffman. "Combining Pharmacological and Cognitive Behavioral Therapy in the Treatment of Anxiety Disorders." In *Oxford Handbook of Anxiety and Related Disorders*, edited by Martin M. Antony and Murray B. Stein, 429–40. New York: Oxford University Press, 2009.

5. Busch, F.N., and B. Milrod. "Psychodynamic Treatment of Panic Disorder." In *Handbook of Evidence-Based Psychodynamic Psychotherapy: Bridging the Gap between Science and Practice*, edited by R. A. Levy and J. S. Ablon, 29–44. Totowa, NJ: Humana Press, 2009.

6. Katzelnick, David J. "Psychopharmacology." In *Helpful Highlights from Heartsome Heedful Headliners*, 1–3. Audio CD. Madison, WI: Audio-Digest Psychiatry, 2008.

7. Krupitsky, E., and E. Kolp. "Ketamine Psychedelic Psychotherapy." In *Psychedelic Medicine: New Evidence for Hallucinogenic Substances as Treatments*, edited by Michael J. Windekman and Thomas B. Roberts, 67–85. Westport, CT: Praeger Publishers/Greenwood Publishing Group, 2007.

8. American College of Obstetricians and Gynecologists. "ACOG Practice Bulletin: Use of Psychiatric Medications during Pregnancy and Lactation." *Obstetrics and Gynecology* 111, no. 4 (2008): 1001–20.

9. Barrett, P., and L. Farrell. "Prevention of Child and Youth Anxiety and Anxiety Disorders." In *Oxford Handbook of Anxiety and Related Disorders*, edited by Martin M. Antony and Murray B. Stein, 497–511. New York: Oxford University Press, 2009.

10. National Institute of Mental Health. *Anxiety Disorders*. Washington, DC: National Institute of Mental Health, 2009.

11. Swartz, K.L. "Depression and Anxiety." In *The Johns Hopkins White Papers*. Baltimore: Johns Hopkins Medical School, 2008.

12. McCabe, R.E., and S. Gifford. "Psychological Treatment of Panic Disorder and Agoraphobia." In *Handbook of Anxiety and Related Disorders*, edited by Martin M. Antony and Murray B. Stein, 308–20. New York: Oxford University Press, 2009.

13. Norton, P.J. "Integrated Psychological Treatment of Multiple Anxiety Disorders." In *Oxford Handbook of Anxiety and Related Disorders*, edited by Martin M. Antony and Murray B. Stein, 441–50. New York: Oxford University Press, 2009.

14. Moskovitch, D.A., M.M. Antony, and R.P. Swinson. "Exposure-Based Treatments for Anxiety Disorders: Theory and Process." In *Oxford Handbook of Anxiety and Related Disorders*, edited by Martin M. Antony and Murray B. Stein, 461–75. New York: Oxford University Press, 2009.

15. Stewart, R. E., and D. L. Chambless. "Cognitive-Behavioral Therapy for Adult Anxiety Disorders in Clinical Practice: A Meta-Analysis of Effectiveness Studies." *Journal of Consulting and Clinical Psychology* 77 (2009): 595–606.

16. Van Ingen, D.J., S.R. Freiheit, and C.S. Vye. "From the Lab to the Clinic: Effectiveness of Cognitive-Behavioral Treatments for Anxiety Disorders." *Professional Psychology: Research and Practice* 40, no. 1 (2009): 69–74.

17. Steward, R.E. "Cognitive-Behavioral Therapy for Adult Anxiety Disorders in Clinical Practice: A Meta-Analysis of Effectiveness Studies." *Journal of Consulting and Clinical Psychology* 77 (2009): 595–606.

18. Marks, I.M. *Fears, Phobias, and Rituals*. New York: Oxford University Press, 1987.

19. Rothbaum, B.O., E.A. Meadows, P. Resick, and D.W. Foy. "Cognitive-Behavioral Therapy." In *Effective Treatments for PTSD: Practice Guidelines from the International Society for Traumatic Stress Studies*, edited by M.J. Friedman, 320–25. New York: Guilford Press, 2000.

20. MacLeod, C., E.H. W. Koster, and E. Fox. "Whither Cognitive Bias Modification Research? Commentary on the Special Section Articles." *Journal of Abnormal Psychology* 118, no. 1 (2009): 89–99.

21. Siev, J. "Specificity of Treatment Effects: Cognitive Therapy and Relaxation for Generalized Anxiety and Panic Disorders." *Journal of Consulting and Clinical Psychology* 75, no. 4 (2007): 513–22.

22. Tryon, W.W., and J.R. Misurell. "Dissonance Induction and Reduction: A Possible Principle and Connectionist Mechanism for Why Therapies Are Effective." *Clinical Psychology Review* 28, no. 8 (2008): 1297–1309.

23. Wood, J.J., and B.D. McLeod, eds. *Child Anxiety Disorders: A Family-Based Treatment Manual for Practitioners*. New York: Norton, 2008.

24. Carr, Alan. "The Effectiveness of Family Therapy and Systemic Interventions for Adult-Focused Problems." *Journal of Family Therapy* 31, no. 1 (2009): 46–74.

25. Ollendick, T.H., L-G. Ost, L. Reuterskiold, N. Costa, R. Cederland, S. Sirbu, T.E. Davis, III, and M.A. Jarrett. "One-Session Treatment of Specific Phobias in Youth: A Randomized Clinical Trial in the United States and Sweden." *Journal of Consulting and Clinical Psychology* 77, no. 3 (2009): 504–16.

26. Eagle, J.L. "Engaging the 'Wise Mind' of a Teen: Incorporating Mindfulness Practice into a Group Therapy Protocol for Anxious Adolescents." Working Paper. Massachusetts School of Professional Psychology, 2009.

27. Reger, M.A., and G.A. Gahm. "A Meta-Analysis of the Effects of Internet- and Computer-Based Cognitive-Behavioral Treatments for Anxiety." *Journal of Clinical Psychology* 65, no. 1 (2009): 53–75.

28. First, M.B., and A. Tasman. "Anxiety Disorders: Social and Specific Phobias." In *DSM-IV-TR Mental Disorders: Diagnosis, Etiology, and Treatment*, edited by M.B. First and A. Tasman, 867–901. Chichester, England: John Wiley, 2004.

29. Clinician's Research Digest. "Using EMDR to Treat Psychological Trauma." *Clinician's Research Digest*. Washington, DC: American Psychological Association, 1997.

30. Lee, C.W., and S. Schubert. "Omissions and Errors in the Institute of Medicine's Report on Scientific Evidence of Treatment for Posttraumatic Stress Disorder." *Journal of EMDR Practice and Research* 3, no. 1 (2009): 32–38.

31. Rogers, C.R. *On Becoming a Person*. New York: Houghton Mifflin, 1961.

32. Roemer, L., S.M. Erisman, and S.M. Orsillo. "Mindfulness and Acceptance-Based Treatments for Anxiety Disorders." In *Oxford Handbook of Anxiety and Related Disorders*, edited by Martin M. Antony and Murray B. Stein, 476–87. New York: Oxford University Press, 2009.

33. Clark, L.A., and D. Watson. "Tripartite Model of Anxiety and Depression: Psychometric Evidence and Taxonomic Implications." *Journal of Abnormal Psychology* 100, no. 3 (1991): 316–36.

34. Pull, C.B. "Current Empirical Status of Acceptance and Commitment Therapy." *Current Opinion in Psychiatry* 22, no. 1 (2009): 55–60.

35. Arch, J.J., and M.G. Craske. "Acceptance and Commitment Therapy and Cognitive Behavioral Therapy for Anxiety Disorders: Different Treatments, Similar Mechanisms?" *Clinical Psychology: Science and Practice* 15, no. 4 (2008): 263–79.

36. Wilkniss, S., and K. Davis. "Review of Trauma, Recovery and Growth: Positive Psychological Perspectives on Posttraumatic Stress." *Psychiatric Rehabilitation Journal* 32, no. 3 (2009): 241–42.

37. Norton, P. "An Open Trial of a Transdiagnostic Cognitive-Behavioral Group Therapy for Anxiety Disorders." *Behavior Therapy* 39, no. 3 (2008): 242–50.

CHAPTER 8

1. Swartz, K. "Depression and Anxiety." In *The Johns Hopkins White Papers*. Baltimore: Johns Hopkins Medical School, 2007.

2. "Combination Therapy for Panic Disorder." *Harvard Mental Health Letter*. Boston: Harvard Medical School, 2008.

3. Uhlenhuth, E.H., M.B. Balter, T.A. Ban, and K. Yang. "International Study of Expert Judgment on Therapeutic Use of Benzodiazepines and Other Psychotherapeutic Medications: VI. Trends in Recommendations for the Pharmacotherapy of Anxiety Disorders, 1992–1997." *Depression and Anxiety* 9 (1999): 107–16.

4. Lader, M.H. "Limitations on the Use of Benzodiazepines in Anxiety and Insomnia: Are They Justified?" *European Neuropsychopharmacology* 9, Suppl. 6 (1999): S399–S405.

5. Ballenger, J.C., J.R.T. Davidson, Y. Lecrubier, D.J. Nutt, T.D. Borkovec, K. Rickels, K.J. Stein, and H-U. Wittchen. "Consensus Statement on Generalized Anxiety Disorder from the International Consensus on Depression and Anxiety." *Journal of Clinical Psychiatry* 62, Suppl. 11 (2001): 53–58.

6. Brawman-Mintzer, O., and R.B. Lydiard. "Psychopharmacology of Anxiety Disorders." *Psychiatric Clinics of North America* 1 (1994): 51–79.

7. Rickels, K., W.G. Case, R.W. Downing, and R. Fridman. "One-Year Follow-up of Anxious Patients Treated with Diazepam." *Journal of Clinical Psychopharmacology* 6 (1986): 32–35.

8. Allgulander, C., D. Hackett, and E. Salinas. "Venlafaxine Extended Release (ER) in the Treatment of Generalized Anxiety Disorder." *British Journal of Psychiatry* 179 (2001): 15–22.

9. Roemer, L., S.M. Orsillo, and K. Salters-Pednealt. "Efficacy of an Acceptance-Based Behavior Therapy for Generalized Anxiety Disorder: Evaluation in a Randomized Controlled Trial." *Journal of Consulting and Clinical Psychology* 76, no. 6 (2008): 1083–89.

10. Amir, N., C. Beard, M. Burns, and J. Bomyea. "Attention Modification Program in Individuals with Generalized Anxiety Disorder." *Journal of Abnormal Psychology* 118, no. 1 (2009): 28–33.

11. "Treating Social Anxiety Disorder." *Harvard Mental Health Letter*. Boston: Harvard Medical School, 2010.

12. WebMD. "Social Anxiety Disorder: Treatment Overview." (2007), http://www.webmd.com/anxiety-panic/tc/social-anxiety-disorder-treatment-overview.

13. Herbert, J.D., B.A. Gaudiano, A.A. Rheingold, E. Moitra, V.H. Myers, K.L. Dalrymple, and L.L. Brandsma. "Cognitive Behavior Therapy for Generalized Social Anxiety Disorder in Adolescents: A Randomized Controlled Trial." *Journal of Anxiety Disorders* 23, no. 2 (2009): 167–77.

14. McManus, F., D.M. Clark, N. Grey, J. Wild, C. Hirsch, M. Fennell, A. Hackmann, L. Waddington, S. Liness, and J. Manley. "A Demonstration of the Efficacy of Two of the Components of Cognitive Therapy for Social Phobia." *Journal of Anxiety Disorders* 23, no. 4 (2009): 496–503.

15. Aderka, I.M. "Factors Affecting Treatment Efficacy in Social Phobia: The Use of Video Feedback and Individual vs. Group Formats." *Journal of Anxiety Disorders* 23, no. 1 (2009): 12–17.

16. First, M.B., and A. Tasman. *DSM-IV-TR Mental Disorders: Diagnosis, Etiology, and Treatment*. Hoboken, NJ: John Wiley, 2004.

17. "Treating Obsessive-Compulsive Disorder." *Harvard Mental Health Letter*. Boston: Harvard Medical School, 2009.

18. Koran, L.M., F.R. Sallee, and S. Pallanti. "Rapid Benefit of Intravenous Pulse Loading of Clomipramine in Obsessive-Compulsive Disorder." *American Journal of Psychiatry* 154 (1997): 396–401.

19. Jenike, M.A. "Augmentation Strategies for Treatment-Resistant Obsessive-Compulsive Disorder." *Harvard Review of Psychiatry* 1 (1993): 17–26.

20. Jenike, M.A. "Pharmacologic Treatment of Obsessive-Compulsive Disorders." *Psychiatric Clinics of North America* 15 (1992): 895–919.

21. McCabe, R.E., and S. Gifford. "Psychological Treatment of Panic Disorder and Agoraphobia." In *Handbook of Anxiety and Related Disorders*, edited by Martin M. Antony and Murray B. Stein, 308–20. New York: Oxford University Press, 2009.

22. Greist, J.H. "Behavior Therapy for Obsessive-Compulsive Disorder." *Journal of Clinical Psychiatry* 55, Suppl. (1994): 36–43.

23. Donahue, C.B. "Impulsivity, Addiction, and OCD." In *7th Annual Psychiatry Review: The Impulsive-Compulsive Spectrum*. Audio CD. University of Minnesota Medical School: Audio-Digest Psychiatry, 2007.

24. Simpson, H.B., K.S. Garfinkle, and M.R. Liebowitz. "Cognitive-Behavioral Therapy as an Adjunct to Serotonin Reuptake Inhibitors in Obsessive-Compulsive Disorder: An Open Trial." *Journal of Clinical Psychiatry* 60 (1999): 584–90.

25. Direnfeld, D., M.T. Pato, and S. Gunn. "Behavior Therapy as Adjuvant Treatment in OCD." Paper presented at the American Psychological Association Annual Meeting. Chicago, 2000.

26. O'Sullivan, G., and I. Marks. "Follow-up Studies of Behavioral Treatment of Phobia and Obsessive-Compulsive Neurosis." *Psychiatric Annals* 21 (1991): 368–73.

27. Nakatani, E., D. Mataix-Cols, N. Micali, C. Turner, and I. Heyman. "Outcomes of Cognitive Behavior Therapy for Obsessive Compulsive Disorder in a Clinical Setting: A 10-Year Experience from a Specialist OCD Service for Children and Adolescents." *Child and Adolescent Mental Health* 14 (2009): 133–39.

28. Whittal, M.L., M. Robichaud, D.S. Thordarson, and P.D. McLean. "Group and Individual Treatment of Obsessive-Compulsive Disorder Using Cognitive Ther-

apy and Exposure Plus Response Prevention: A 2-Year Follow-up of Two Randomized Trials." *Journal of Consulting and Clinical Psychology* 76, no. 6 (2008): 1003–14.

29. Andres, S., L. Lazaro, M. Salamero, T. Boget, R. Penades, and J. Castro. "Changes in Cognitive Dysfunction in Children and Adolescents with Obsessive-Compulsive Disorder after Treatment." *Journal of Psychiatric Research* 42, no. 6 (2008): 507–14.

30. Schoenfeld, F. "Posttraumatic Stress Disorder: Part 2." In *PTSD: In an Age of Violence, Terror, and Disaster*. Audio CD. San Francisco: Audio-Digest Psychiatry, 2008.

31. Mansell, P., and J. Read. "Post-Traumatic Stress Disorder, Drug Companies, and the Internet." *Journal of Trauma and Dissociation* 10, no. 1 (2009): 9–23.

32. Serretti, A., A. Chiesa, R. Calati, G. Perna, L. Bellodi, and D. De Ronchi. "Common Genetic, Clinical, Demographic, and Psychosocial Predictors of Response to Pharmacotherapy in Mood and Anxiety Disorders." *International Clinical Psychopharmacology* 24, no. 1 (2009): 1–18.

33. Muris, P., B. Mayer, M. den Adel, T. Roos, and J. van Wamelen. "Predictors of Change Following Cognitive-Behavioral Treatment of Children with Anxiety Problems: A Preliminary Investigation on Negative Automatic Thoughts and Anxiety Control." *Child Psychiatry and Human Development* 40, no. 1 (2009): 139–51.

34. Ollendick, T. H., L-G. Ost, L. Reuterskiold, N. Costa, R. Cederland, S. Sirbu, Davis III T. E., and M. A. Jarrett. "One-Session Treatment of Specific Phobias in Youth: A Randomized Clinical Trial in the United States and Sweden." *Journal of Consulting and Clinical Psychology* 77, no. 3 (2009): 504–16.

35. Kendall, P. C. "In-Session Exposure Tasks and Therapeutic Alliance across the Treatment of Childhood Anxiety Disorders." *Journal of Consulting and Clinical Psychology* 77, no. 3 (2009): 517–25.

36. Ginsburg, G. S. "The Child Anxiety Prevention Study: Intervention Model and Primary Outcomes." *Journal of Consulting and Clinical Psychology* 77, no. 3 (2009): 580–87.

37. Wood, J. J., A. W. Chiu, H. Wei-Chin, J. Jacobs, and M. Ifekwunigwe. "Adapting Cognitive-Behavioral Therapy for Mexican American Students with Anxiety Disorders: Recommendations for School Psychologists." *School Psychology Quarterly* 23, no. 4 (2008): 515–32.

38. Montgomery, S., K. Chatamra, E. Whelen, and F. Baldinette. "Efficacy and Safety of Pregabalin in Elderly People with Generalized Anxiety Disorder." *British Journal of Psychiatry* 193, no. 5 (2008): 389–94.

39. Healthy Place. "Anxiety in the Elderly." *HealthyPlace.com* (2007), http://www.healthyplace.com/anxiety-panic/main/anxiety-in-the-elderly.html.

CHAPTER 10

1. Yates, William R. "Somatoform Disorders." *EMedicine* (2008), http://emedicine.medscape.com/article/294908-print.

2. First, M. B., and A. Tasman. *DSM-IV-TR Mental Disorders: Diagnosis, Etiology, and Treatment*. Hoboken, NJ: John Wiley, 2004.

3. Malt, U. F. "Somatization: An Old Disorder in New Bottles." *Psychiatrica Fennica* 22 (1991): 1–13.

4. Parsons, Talcott. *The Social Structure*. Glencoe, IL: Free Press, 1951.

5. Feldman, M. "Factitious Disorders." In *Comprehensive Textbook of Psychiatry*, 7th ed., edited by B. Sadock and V. Sadock, 1533–44. Philadelphia: Lippincott, Williams & Wilkins, 2000.

6. Asher, R. "Munchausen's Syndrome." *Lancet* 1 (1951): 339–41.

7. Wise, M. G., and C. V. Ford. "Factitious Disorders." *Primary Care* 26, no. 2 (1999): 315–26.

8. Plassman, R. "Munchausen's Syndrome and Factitious Diseases." *Psychotherapy and Psychosomatics* 62, no. 1–2 (1994): 7–26.

9. Goldstein, A. B. "Identification and Classification of Factitious Disorders: An Analysis of Cases Reported during a Ten-Year Period." *International Journal of Psychiatry in Medicine* 28, no. 2 (1998): 221–41.

10. Ehlers, W., and R. Plassman. "Diagnosis of Narcissistic Self-Esteem Regulation in Patients with Factitious Illness (Munchausen Syndrome)." *Psychotherapy and Psychosomatics* 62 (1994): 69–77.

11. Kent, J. D. "Munchausen's Syndrome and Substance Abuse." *Journal of Substance Abuse Treatment* 11, no. 3 (1994): 247–51.

12. McKane, J. P., and J. Anderson. "Munchausen's Syndrome: Rule Breakers and Risk Takers." *British Journal of Hospital Medicine* 58, no. 4 (1997): 150–53.

13. Eisendrath, S. J. "Factitious Disorders and Malingering." In *Treatment of Psychiatric Disorders*, 3rd. ed., edited by G. O. Gabbard, 1825–44. Washington, DC: American Psychiatric Publishing, 2001.

14. Breuer, Josef, and Sigmund Freud. "Studies on Hysteria." In *The Standard Edition of the Complete Psychological Works of Sigmund Freud*, edited by J. Strachy (trans. ed.). London: Hogarth Press (originally published in 1893–1895), 1955.

15. American Psychiatric Association. *Diagnostic and Statistical Manual, Fourth Edition, Text Revision*. Washington, DC: American Psychiatric Association, 2000.

16. Phillips, K. A. "Somatization Disorder." (2008),. http://www.merckmanuals.com/professional/sec16/ch214/ch214g.html.

17. Maloney, M. J. "Diagnosing Hysterical Conversion Disorders in Children." *Journal of Pediatrics* 97 (1980): 1016–20.

18. Weddington, W. W. "Conversion Reaction in an 82-Year-Old Man." *Journal of Nervous and Mental Disease* 167 (1979): 368–69.

19. Tomasson, K., D. Kent, and W. Coryell. "Somatization and Conversion Disorders: Comorbidity and Demographics at Presentation." *Acta Psychiatrica Scandinavia* 84 (1991): 288–93.

20. Lewis, W. C., and M. Berman. "Studies of Conversion Hysteria. I. Operational Study of Diagnosis." *Archives of General Psychiatry* 13 (1965): 275–82.

21. Weinstein, E. A., R. A. Eck, and O. G. Lyerly. "Conversion Hysteria in Appalachia." *Psychiatry* 32 (1969): 334–41.

22. Raskin, M., J. A. Talbott, and A. T. Meyerson. "Diagnosis of Conversion Reactions: Predictive Value of Psychiatric Criteria." *Journal of the American Medical Association* 197 (1966): 530–34.

23. Lewis, W. C. "Hysteria: The Consultant's Dilemma: 20th Century Demonology, Pejorative Epithet, or Useful Diagnosis." *Archives of General Psychiatry* 30 (1974): 145–51.

24. Toone, B. K. "Disorders of Hysterical Conversion." In *Physical Symptoms and Psychological Illness*, edited by C. Bass, 207–34. London: Blackwell Scientific, 1990.

25. Ford, C.V. "Conversion Disorder and Somatoform Disorder Not Otherwise Specified." In *Treatments of Psychiatric Disorders*, vol. 2, 2nd ed., edited by G.O. Gabbard, 1735–53. Washington, DC: American Psychiatric Association, 1995.

26. Cloninger, C.R., R.L. Martin, S.B. Guze, and P.J. Clayton. "A Prospective Follow-up and Family Study of Somatization in Men and Women." *American Journal of Psychiatry* 143 (1986): 873–78.

27. Martin, R.L. "Problems in the Diagnosis of Somatization Disorder: Effects on Research and Clinical Practice." *Psychiatric Annals* 18 (1988): 357–62.

28. King, S.A. "Pain Disorders." In *The American Psychiatric Press Textbook of Psychiatry*, 2nd ed., edited by R.E. Hales, S.C. Yudofsky and J.A. Talbott, 591–622. Washington, DC: American Psychiatric Press, 1994.

29. Osterweis, M., A. Kleinman, and D. Mechanic, eds. *Pain and Disability*. Washington, DC: National Academy Press, 1987.

30. Andreasen, N.C., and J. Bardach. "Dysmorphobphobia: Symptom or Disease." *American Journal of Psychiatry* 134 (1977): 673–76.

31. Phillips, K.A., S.L. McElroy Jr., P.E. Peck Jr., H.G. Pope, and J.I. Hudson. "Body Dysmorphic Disorder: 30 Cases of Imagined Ugliness." *American Journal of Psychiatry* 150 (1993): 302–8.

CHAPTER 11

1. Sadock, B., and V. Sadock. *Kaplan and Sadock's Synopsis of Psychiatry: Behavioral Sciences/Clinical Psychiatry*, 9th ed. Philadelphia: Lippincott, Williams, & Wilkins, 2002.

2. Atchison, M., and A.C. McFarlane. "A Review of Dissociation and Dissociative Disorders." *Australian and New Zealand Journal of Psychiatry* 28, no. 4 (1994): 591–99.

3. Rieber, R.W. "The Duality of the Brain and the Multiplicity of Minds: Can You Have It Both Ways?" *History of Psychiatry* 13, no. 49 Pt. 1 (2002): 3–17.

4. Borch-Jacobson, M., and D. Brick. "How to Predict the Past: From Trauma to Repression." *History of Psychiatry* 11, no. 11 Pt. 1 (2000): 15–35.

5. Janet, Pierre. *The Major Symptoms of Hysteria*. New York: Macmillan, 1920.

6. van der Kolk, B.A., and O. van der Hart. "Pierre Janet and the Breakdown of Adaptation in Psychological Trauma." *American Journal of Psychiatry* 146, no. 12 (1989): 1530–40.

7. Putnam, F.W. *Diagnosis and Treatment of Multiple Personality Disorder*. New York: Guilford Press, 1989.

8. First, M.B., and A. Tasman. *DSM-IV-TR Mental Disorders: Diagnosis, Etiology, and Treatment*. Hoboken, NJ: John Wiley, 2004.

9. Breuer, J., and S. Freud. "Studies on Hysteria." In *The Standard Edition of the Complete Psychological Works of Sigmund Freud*, edited by J. Strachy (trans. ed.). London: Hogarth Press (originally published in 1893–1895), 1955.

10. Bowman, E.S. "Treatments for Dissociative Disorders." In *Psychiatric Illness in Women: Emerging Treatments and Research*, edited by F. Lewis-Hall, T.S. Williams, J.A. Panetta and J.M. Herrera, 535–55. Arlington, VA: American Psychiatric Publishing, 2002.

11. Schachter, D. "Understanding Implicit Memory: A Cognitive Neuroscience Approach." *American Psychologist* 47 (1992): 559–69.

12. Squire, L. R. *Memory and Brain.* New York: Oxford University Press, 1987.

13. Tulving, E. *Elements of Episodic Memory.* Oxford, England: Clarendon Press, 1983.

14. Kosslyn, S. M., and O. Koenig. *Wet Mind: The New Cognitive Neuroscience.* New York: Free Press, 1992.

15. Spiegel, D., and E. Cardena. "Disintegrated Experience: The Dissociative Disorders Revisited." *Journal of Abnormal Psychology* 100 (1991): 366–78.

16. Coons, P. M., and V. Milstein. "Psychosexual Disturbances in Multiple Personality: Characteristics, Etiology, Treatment." *Journal of Clinical Psychiatry* 47 (1986): 106–10.

17. Coons, P. M. "The Differential Diagnosis of Multiple Personality." *Psychiatric Clinics of North America* 12 (1984): 51–67.

18. Kluft, R. P. "Multiple Personality Disorder." In *American Psychiatric Press Review of Psychiatry,* edited by A. Tasman and S. M. Goldfinger, 161–88. Washington, DC: American Psychiatric Press, 1991.

19. Ross, C. A. "Epidemiology of Multiple Personality Disorder and Dissociation." *Psychiatric Clinics of North America* 14 (1991): 503–18.

20. Schultz, R., B. G. Braun, and R. P. Kluft. "Multiple Personality Disorder: Phenomenology of Selected Variables in Comparison to Jamor Depression." *Dissociation* 2 (1989): 45–51.

21. Saxe, G. N., B. A. van der Kolk, R. Berkowitz, G. Chinman, K. Hall, G. Lieberg, and J. Schwartz. "Dissociative Disorders in Psychiatric Patients." *American Journal of Psychiatry* 150 (1993): 1037–42.

22. Saxena, S., and K. Prasad. "DSM-III Subclassification of Dissociative Disorders Applied to Psychiatric Outpatients in India." *American Journal of Psychiatry* 146 (1989): 261–62.

23. Steinberg, M. "The Spectrum of Depersonalization: Assessment and Treatment." In *American Psychiatric Press Review of Psychiatry,* edited by A. Tasman and S. M. Goldfinger, 233–47. Washington, DC: American Psychiatric Press, 1991.

24. Mayo Clinic. "Dissociative Disorders." *MayoClinic.com* (2009), http://www.mayoclinic.com/health/dissociative-disorders/DS00574/DSECTION=symptoms.

25. Loewenstein, R. J. "Psychogenic Amnesia and Psychogenic Fugue: A Comprehensive Review." In *American Psychiatric Press Review of Psychiatry,* edited by A. Tasman and S. M. Goldfinger, 189–222. Washington, DC: American Psychiatric Press, 1991.

26. Schachter, D. L. "Memory Distortion: History and Current Status." In *Memory Distortion: How Minds, Brains, and Societies Reconstruct the Past,* edited by D. L. Schachter, 1–42. Cambridge, MA: Harvard University Press, 1995.

27. American Psychiatric Association. *Diagnostic and Statistical Manual, Fourth Edition, Text Revision.* Washington, DC: American Psychiatric Association, 2000.

28. Putnam, F. W. *Diagnosis and Treatment of Multiple Personality Disorder.* New York: Guilford Press, 1989.

29. Spiegel, H., and D. Spiegel. *Trance and Treatment: Clinical Uses of Hypnosis.* New York: Harper-Collins, 1978.

30. Spiegel, D. "Vietnam Grief Work Using Hypnosis." *American Journal of Clinical Hypnosis* 24 (1981): 33–40.

31. Kirmayer, K. J. "Pacing the Void: Social and Cultural Dimensions of Dissociation." In *Dissociation: Culture, Mind and Body*, edited by D. Spiegel, 91–122. Washington, DC: American Psychiatric Press, 1994.

32. Lewis-Fernandez, R. "Culture and Dissociation: A Comparison of Ataque de Nervios among Puerto Ricans and 'Possession Syndrome' In India." In *Dissociation: Culture, Mind and Body*, edited by D. Spiegel, 123–67. Washington, DC: American Psychiatric Press, 1994.

33. Spanos, Nicholas P., John R. Weekes, and Lorne D. Bertrand. "Multiple Personality Disorder: A Social Psychological Perspective." *Journal of Abnormal Psychology* 94, no. 3 (1985): 362–76.

34. Putnam, F. W., J. J. Guroff, E. K. Silberman, L. Barban, and R. M. Post. "The Clinical Phenomenology of Multiple Personality Disorder: Review of 100 Recent Cases." *Journal of Clinical Psychiatry* 47 (1986): 285–93.

35. Mayo Clinic. "Dissociative Disorders." *MayoClinic.com* (2009), http://www.mayoclinic.com/health/dissociative-disorders/DS00574/DSECTION=symptoms.

36. Boon, S., and N. Draijer. "Multiple Personality Disorder in the Netherlands: A Clinical Investigation of 71 Patients." *American Journal of Psychiatry* 150 (1993): 489–94.

37. Ganaway, G. K. "Hypnosis, Childhood Trauma, and Dissociative Identity Disorder, toward an Integrative Theory." *International Journal of Clinical and Experimental Hypnosis* 43 (1995): 127–44.

38. Ross, C. A., S. D. Miller, P. Reagor, L. Bjornson, G. A. Fraser, and G. Anderson. "Structured Interview Data on 102 Cases of Multiple Personality Disorder from Four Centers." *American Journal of Psychiatry* 147 (1990): 596–601.

39. Spiegel, D. "Chronic Pain Masks Depression, Multiple Personality Disorder." *Hospital and Community Psychiatry* 38 (1987): 933–35.

40. Piper, A., and H. Merskey. "The Persistence of Folly: A Critical Examination of Dissociative Identity Disorder. Part 1. The Excesses of an Improbable Concept." *Canadian Journal of Psychiatry* 49 (2004): 592–600.

41. Thigpen, G. H., and H. M. Cleckley. "On the Incidence of Multiple Personality Disorder: A Brief Communication." *International Journal of Clinical and Experimental Hypnosis* 32 (1984): 64.

42. Maldonado, J. R., and D. Spiegel. "Dissociative States." In *The American Psychiatric Publishing Textbook of Personality Disorders*, edited by J. M. Oldham, A. E. Skodol, and D. S. Bender, 492–521. Arlington, VA: American Psychiatric Publishing, 2005.

43. Nijenhuis, E.R.S., P. Spinhoven, R. van Dyck, O. van der Hart, and J. Vanderlinden. "Degree of Somatoform and Psychological Dissociation in Dissociative Disorders Is Correlated with Reported Trauma." *Journal of Traumatic Stress* 11 (1998): 711–30.

44. Chu, J. A., and D. L. Dill. "Dissociative Symptoms in Relation to Childhood Physical and Sexual Abuse." *American Journal of Psychiatry* 146, no. 7 (1990): 887–92.

45. Demitrack, M. A., F. M. Putnam, T. D. Brewerton, H. A. Brandt, and P. W. Gold. "Relation of Clinical Variables to Dissociative Phenomena in Eating Disorders." *American Journal of Psychiatry* 147 (1990): 1184–88.

46. Bremner, J. D., J. H. Krystal, D. S. Charney, and S. M. Southwick. "Neural Mechanisms in Dissociative Amnesia for Childhood Abuse: Relevance to the Current Controversy Surrounding the 'False Memory Syndrome.'" *American Journal of Psychiatry* 153 (1996): 71–82.

47. Maldonado, J. R., L. D. Butler, and D. Spiegel. "Treatment of Dissociative Disorders." In *Treatments That Work*, edited by P. Nathan and J. M. Gorman, 463–96. New York: Oxford University Press, 2000.

48. Simon, N. M., R. E. Kaufman, E. A. Hoge, J. J. Worthington, N. N. Herlands, M. E. Owens, and M. H. Pollack. "Open-Label Support for Duloxetine for the Treatment of Panic Disorder." *CNS: Neuroscience and Therapeutics* 15, no. 1 (2009): 19–23.

49. Kluft, R. C. "Reflections on the Traumatic Memories of Dissociative Identity Disorder Patients." In *Truth in Memory*, edited by S. J. Lynn and K. M. McConkey, 304–22. New York: Guilford Press, 1996.

50. Kluft, R. P. "An Overview of the Psychotherapy of Dissociative Identity Disorder." *American Journal of Psychotherapy* 53, no. 3 (1999): 289–319.

51. Loewenstein, R. J. "Psychopharmacologic Treatments for Dissociative Identity Disorder." *Psychiatric Annals* 35, no. 8 (2005): 666–73.

52. Maldonado, J. R., and D. Spiegel. "Dissociative States." In *The American Psychiatric Publishing Textbook of Personality Disorders*, edited by J. M. Oldham, A. E. Skodol, and D. S. Bender, 492–521. Arlington, VA: American Psychiatric Publishing, 2005.

Index

ABPP. *See* American Board of Professional Psychology (ABPP)

Acceptance and commitment therapy (ACT), 122–23

Acceptance-based behavior therapy, 127

ACSW. *See* Associate clinical social worker (ACSW)

ACT. *See* Acceptance and commitment therapy (ACT)

Acute Stress Disorder (ASD), 6, 96–97; course of, 97; diagnostic criteria for, 96–97; overview of, 96; treatments for, 133

Advanced practice registered nurse (APRN), 142

African Americans, anxiety and, 40–41

Age of Anxiety, 2–4

Agoraphobia, 6, 85; African Americans and, 40; biological theories for, 51; diagnostic criteria for, 79; gender and, 31; Panic Disorder and, 78, 79; physical factors of, 66

Alaskan Natives, anxiety and, 45

Alcohol/drug counselor, 142

American Board of Professional Psychology (ABPP), 144

American Psychiatric Association, 5, 101

American Psychological Association, 56

Amygdala, anxiety development and, 52, 70

Antianxiety (anxiolytic) medications, 111–12

Antidepressant medications, 110–11

Anxiety: African Americans and, 40–41; age and, 32–39; Alaskan Natives and, 45; Asian Americans and, 42–44; causes of, 3; changing conceptions of, 183–86; children and teens and, 32–36; coping strategies for, 187–90; definition of, 1–2; elderly and, 36–39; feelings of, 3–4; Hispanic Americans and, 44–45; homosexual groups and, 46–47; men and, 31–32; myths about, 7–11; Native Americans and, 45; religious groups and, 47; symptoms of, 2; treatment of, 5; women and, 30–31; word origin of, 2

Anxiety Disorder Due to a General Medical Condition, 6

Anxiety Disorder Not Otherwise Specified, 6

Anxiety Disorders. *See also* Anxiety: biological theories of, 49–54; children and, 33; in college students,

34–35; considerations in treating, 135–38; costs associated with, 29–30; course of treatment for, 6; definition of, 2; demographics associated with, 31–32; diagnosing, 4–6; distribution and effects of, 29–48; ethnicity and, 39–46; gender and, 30–32; living with (case studies), 15–28; perceived *vs.* real threat and, 2–3; race and, 39–46; theories of, 49–67; treatments for, 107–23; twins and, 50; well-known people suffering from, 11–13

Anxiety Disorders, living with, 139–50; effects of treatment, 145–47; mental health professional types, 140–45; stress management and, 147–50; where to seek treatment, 140; who needs treatment, 139–40

Anxiety Disorders I, types of, 73–82; Generalized Anxiety Disorder as, 73–76; Panic Disorder as, 76–82

Anxiety Disorders II, types of, 83–105; Acute Stress Disorder as, 96–99; Obsessive-Compulsive Disorder as, 99–105; Phobias as, 83–89; Posttraumatic Stress Disorder as, 89–99

Anxiety-like symptoms, sources of, 72

Anxiety sensitivity model, 62

Anxiolytics, 114

APRN. *See* Advanced practice registered nurse (APRN)

ASD. *See* Acute Stress Disorder (ASD); Autistic Spectrum Disorder (ASD)

Asian Americans, anxiety and, 42–44

Associate clinical social worker (ACSW), 142

Autistic Spectrum Disorder (ASD), 35

Avoidance as Posttraumatic Stress Disorder symptom, 91

Axis, diagnosis and, 6

Bandura, Albert, 60

Basinger, Kim, 69

Battle fatigue, 89

BDD. *See* Body Dysmorphic Disorder (BDD)

Beck, Aaron, 62

Behavioral inhibition system (BIS), 52

Behavioral theorists, 58–61

Behavior inhibition, 61

Benzodiazepines, 113

Beta blockers, 114

Biological theories of Anxiety Disorder, 49–54; central nervous system role and, 52; corticotrophin releasing factor and, 52; genetic contributions role and, 49–51; neurotransmitter systems and, 52–53; serotonin and, 53

BIS. *See* Behavioral inhibition system (BIS)

Body Dysmorphic Disorder (BDD), 165–67; concerns of patients with, 166; diagnostic criteria of, 165; treatment of, 167

Brain, response to stress and anxiety of, 69–70

Breast-feeding and antianxiety medications, 115–16

Breuer, Josef, 160

Catecholamines, 70

CBT. *See* Cognitive-behavioral therapy (CBT)

Charcot, Jean-Martin, 116, 170

Children, anxiety in, 32–36; comorbid conditions and, 35; diagnosing, 32–34; Sleep-Related Problems and, 35; treating, 35–36

Cigarette smoking as Anxiety Disorder risk factor, 53–54

Circulatory system, responses to stress and anxiety of, 70

Clinical social worker (CSW), 142

Cognitive-behavioral therapy (CBT), 36, 109, 116–19

Cognitive bias modification, 63, 120

Cognitive theorists, 61–64

Combat neurosis, 90

Comorbid conditions, 4–5, 6, 35; African Americans and, 41; of Dissocia-

tive Identity Disorder, 177; of Facti-
tious Disorders, 153; of Generalized
Anxiety Disorder, 75; of Obsessive-
Compulsive Disorder, 102–3; of Pain
Disorder, 164; of Panic Disorder, 80;
of Posttraumatic Stress Disorder, 95,
97; recognizing and treating, 135; of
Social Phobia, 88
Compulsions, types of, 102
Conditions of worth, 57
Conjoint Treatment for Posttraumatic
Stress Disorder (PTSD), 99
Conversion Disorder, 160–63; causes
for, 161–62; diagnostic criteria for,
160; onset of, 161; symptoms of, 162;
treatment for, 162–63
Coping and Promoting Strength Pro-
gram (CPSP), 36
Coping strategies for anxiety, 187–90
Cornell Panic-Anxiety Study Group,
66
Corticotrophin releasing factor, 52, 53
Counselor/therapist, 142
CPSP. See Coping and Promoting
Strength Program (CPSP)
CSW. See Clinical social worker
(CSW)

DA. See Dissociative Amnesia (DA)
Depersonalization Disorder (DPD), 173
Derealization, 173
DFD. See Dissociative Fugue Disorder
(DFD)
Diagnostic and Statistical Manual
(DSM), 5–6; DSM-I, 5, 90; DSM-II,
5, 90; DSM-III, 5, 170; DSM-III-R,
5, 76; DSM-IV, 5–6, 92; DSM-V, 6,
94, 186
Diagnostic and Statistical Manual, 4th
Edition, Text Revision (DSM-IV-TR),
5, 6; Body Dysmorphic Disorder
diagnostic criteria, 165; Obsessive-
Compulsive Disorder diagnostic
criteria, 101; Pain Disorder diagnos-
tic criteria, 163–64; Somatization
Disorder diagnostic criteria, 158–59
Diathesis, 39, 51

DID. See Dissociative Identity Disorder
(DID)
Dissociative Amnesia (DA), 173–75;
characteristics of, 174; diagnosis of,
174; treatment for, 174–75
Dissociative Disorders, 169–82;
background and history of, 169–71;
Depersonalization Disorder as, 173;
diagnosing, 172–73; Dissociative
Amnesia as, 173–75; Dissociative
Fugue Disorder as, 175; Dissociative
Identity Disorder, 176–80; Dis-
sociative Trance Disorder as, 176;
epidemiology of, 172; overview of,
171–72; treatments for, 180–82
Dissociative Fugue Disorder (DFD),
175
Dissociative Identity Disorder (DID),
170, 176–80; comorbidities of, 177;
overview of, 176–77; studies on,
178–79
Dissociative Trance Disorder, 176
Distress, 148
Doctor of social work (DSW), 142
Doctor shopping, 78
Dopaminergic system, anxiety and, 53
DPD. See Depersonalization Disorder
(DPD)
DSM. See Diagnostic and Statistical
Manual (DSM)
DSM-IV-TR. See Diagnostic and Statisti-
cal Manual, 4th Edition, Text Revision
(DSM-IV-TR)
DSW. See Doctor of social work (DSW)

Ego, 54–55
Elderly, anxiety disorders in, 36–39;
treatment of, 39, 137–38
Ellis, Albert, 62
EMDR therapy. See Eye movement
desensitization and reprogramming
(EMDR) therapy
Emotional numbing as Posttraumatic
Stress Disorder symptom, 91
Epidemiologic Catchment Area Study,
40, 85, 93, 103
Eustress, 148

Exercise as stress management strategy, 149

Existential theorists, 56–58

Eye movement desensitization and re-programming (EMDR) therapy, 122

Factitious Disorders, 152–55; comorbid conditions of, 153; diagnosing difficulties with, 154; epidemiology of, 153–54; etiology of, 154; treating, 154–55

FDA. *See* Food and Drug Administration (FDA)

Fight-or-flight reaction, 1, 52, 70

Folate deficiency, anxiety-like symptoms of, 72

Food and Drug Administration (FDA), 114

Frankenstein (Shelley), 170

Frankl, Victor, 57

Freud, Sigmund, 54–56, 116

Fugue state, 175

Functionally autonomous, 9

GABA. *See* Gamma-aminobutyric acid (GABA)

GAD. *See* Generalized Anxiety Disorder (GAD)

Gamma-aminobutyric acid (GABA), 52

Gastrointestinal disease, anxiety-like symptoms of, 72

Generalization, phobias and, 60

Generalized Anxiety Disorder (GAD), 6, 73–76. *See also* Physical responses to stress and anxiety; biological theories for, 51; characteristics of, 73, 74; children with, 34, 75; comorbid conditions of, 75; diagnosis of, 73, 74–75; elderly and, 37; in lesbian and bisexual women, 46; lifetime prevalence rate of, 73; physical symptoms of, 75; treatments for, 76, 126–27

Genotype, 51

Gross stress reaction, 90

Guilt, 55

Heart, responses to stress and anxiety of, 70

Hispanic Americans, anxiety and, 44–45

Homeostatic, 72

Homosexual groups, anxiety and, 46–47

HPA. *See* Hypothalamic-pituitary-adrenal axis (HPA)

Humanistic theorists, 56–58

Hyperarousal as Posttraumatic Stress Disorder symptom, 90

Hyperthyroidism, anxiety-like symptoms of, 72

Hypnosis as Anxiety Disorder treatment, 121–22

Hypochondriasis, 155–58; diagnosing, 155–57; environmental and cultural factors of, 157; treating, 157–58

Hypothalamic-pituitary-adrenal axis (HPA), 52, 69

ICT. *See* Internet and computer-based therapy (ICT)

Immune system, responses to stress and anxiety of, 70

Impulse Control Disorders, 103–4

Infectious disease, anxiety-like symptoms of, 72

Innate valuing tendency, 57

Insomnia and Anxiety Disorders, 54, 66

Institute of Medicine (IOM), 122

Internet and computer-based therapy (ICT), 121

Intrusion as Posttraumatic Stress Disorder symptom, 90–91

IOM. *See* Institute of Medicine (IOM)

Irritable Bowel Syndrome, GAD and, 75

Janet, Pierre, 170

Japanese Americans, anxiety and, 42–43

Kase, Latrina, 107

Kelly, George, 61–62

Kennedy, John F., 29
Kennedy, Rose F., 29
Kundera, Milan, 49

Laing, R. D., 57
LASA. *See* Longitudinal Aging Study
    Amsterdam (LASA)
Latino Paradox, 44
LCSW. *See* Licensed clinical social
    worker (LCSW)
LCSW-R. *See* Licensed clinical social
    worker-R (LCSW-R)
Licensed clinical social worker
    (LCSW), 142
Licensed clinical social worker-R
    (LCSW-R), 142
Limbic system, anxiety development
    and, 52
Little Albert experiment, 58
Longitudinal Aging Study Amsterdam
    (LASA), 37
Loss of control, fear of, 2
Lungs, responses to stress and anxiety
    of, 70

Madden, John, 85
Malingering Disorders, 152–55
MAOIs. *See* Monoamine oxidase
    inhibitors (MAOIs)
Maslow, Abraham, 56
Master's degree in social work (MSW),
    142, 145
Master's of science in nursing (MSN),
    142
May, Rollo, 57
Medical treatments for Anxiety Disor-
    ders, 109–16; antianxiety (anxi-
    olytic) medications for, 111–12;
    antidepressant medications for,
    110–11; drugs and natural substances
    for, 112–15; overview of, 109–10;
    pregnancy and, 115–16
Medications, anxiety-like symptoms
    of, 72
Men and anxiety, 31–32
Menopause, anxiety-like symptoms of,
    72

Mental health professionals, types of,
    140–45
Metabolic responses to stress and
    anxiety, 71
Mexican American youth and Anxiety
    Disorder treatment, 136–37
Mindfulness meditation, 122
Mitral valve prolapse, 66
Monoamine oxidase inhibitors
    (MAOIs), 111
Moral anxiety, 55
Mouth and throat, responses to stress
    and anxiety of, 71
Mowrer, O. H., 59–60
MSN. *See* Master's of science in nursing
    (MSN)
MSW. *See* Master's degree in social
    work (MSW)
Multiaxial diagnoses, 6
Multiple Personality Disorder, 176
Munchausen's Syndrome, 153
Myths about anxiety, 7–11

Narcoanalysis, 163
National Register of Health Service
    Providers in Psychology, 144
Native Americans, anxiety and, 45
Natural substances as medical treat-
    ments for Anxiety Disorders, 114–15
Neurotic anxiety, 55
Nicholson, Jack, 83
Niebuhr, Reinhold, 147
Noradrenergic system, anxiety and, 52
NP. *See* Nurse practitioner (NP)
Nurse practitioner (NP), 141–42
Nutrition and stress management, 150

Observational learning, 60
Obsessions, types of, 101–2
Obsessive-Compulsive Disorder
    (OCD), 6, 99–105; celebrities who
    suffer from, 12; comorbid conditions
    of, 102–3; diagnosing, 100–101,
    103–4; etiology issues with, 104;
    genetic basis for, 51, 104; Impulse
    Control Disorders and, 103–4; living
    with (case study), 15–21; overview

of, 99–100; treatments for, 104–5, 130–33; types of compulsions, 102; types of obsessions, 101–2
Obsessive-Compulsive Personality Disorder (OCPD), 100
OCD. *See* Obsessive-Compulsive Disorder (OCD)
OCPD. *See* Obsessive-Compulsive Personality Disorder (OCPD)

Pain Disorder, 163–65; comorbid conditions of, 164; diagnostic criteria for, 163–64; treating, 164–65
Panic attacks, 76–77, 81–82
Panic Disorder (PD), 6, 30, 76–82. *See also* Physical responses to stress and anxiety; in adolescent, 34, 77; African Americans and, 40, 41; Agoraphobia and, 78, 79; biological theories for, 51; characteristics of, 76–77; comorbid conditions of, 80; diagnosis of, 77–79; in gay and bisexual men, 46; lifetime prevalence rate of, 77–78; panic attacks and, 76–77, 81–82; physical factors of, 66; risk factors for, 80; symptoms of, 78–79; treatments for, 80–81, 125–26
Parsons, Talcott, 152
Partial Posttraumatic Stress Disorder, 92
Patient vulnerability and Anxiety Disorder, 65–67
Pavlov, Ivan, 58–59
PD. *See* Panic Disorder (PD)
Perfectionism, Social Phobia and, 61
Personal construct theory, 61–62
Phobias, 83–89; diagnosis of, 84–85; groups of, 85; Social, 85, 86–89; Specific, 85–86; unusual, 83–84
Physical responses to stress and anxiety, 69–72; brain responses, 69–70; heart, lungs, circulatory system responses, 70; immune system responses, 70; metabolic responses, 71; mouth and throat responses, 71; other sources of symptoms and, 72; skin responses, 71; when stress

or anxiety disappears or continues, 71–72
Pleasure center, 52
Poe, Edgar Alan, 170
Positive voice, being a, 190–92
Posttraumatic Stress Disorder (PTSD), 6, 30, 89–99. *See also* Acute Stress Disorder (ASD); chronic medical conditions and, 66–67; comorbid conditions of, 95, 97; Conjoint Treatment for, 99; course and outlook of, 95–96; defining traumatic and, 93; diagnostic criteria for, 91–92; factors affecting development of, 98; highest risk groups for, 98–99; Korean War and, 90; lifetime prevalence rate of, 91; men *vs.* women and, 93–94; Native American veterans and, 45; other names for, 89–90; overview of, 89–90; reasons for misdiagnosing, 95; symptoms of, 90–91, 92; treatment of, 97–98, 133–35; vulnerability factors to, 94
Pregabalin, 137
Pregnancy and antianxiety medications, 115–16
Psychiatrist, 141, 144
Psychoanalysis, 54
Psychodynamic approaches, 54–56
Psychological theories of Anxiety Disorder, 54–64; behavioral approaches to, 58–61; cognitive approaches to, 61–64; humanistic and existential approaches to, 56–58; psychodynamic approaches to, 54–56
Psychological treatments of Anxiety Disorders, 116–19
Psychologist, 141, 143–44
Psychosocial approaches to Anxiety Disorders, 119–23
Psychosomatic, 152
Psychotherapist, 142
PTSD. *See* Posttraumatic Stress Disorder (PTSD)

Rational-emotive psychotherapy, 62
Reality anxiety, 55

Recreation as stress management strategy, 149

Re-experiencing as Posttraumatic Stress Disorder symptom, 90–91

Reframing, 118

Relaxation as stress management strategy, 149

Relaxation training as Anxiety Disorders treatment, 120

Religious groups, anxiety and, 47

Roche, Arthur Somers, 15

Rogers, Carl, 56; model of anxiety, 57

Rule of Thirds, 181

Rutherford, Mark, 1

SAD. *See* Seasonal Affective Disorder (SAD)

Schemata, 64

Seasonal Affective Disorder (SAD), 80

Selective information processing, 62–63

Selective serotonin reuptake inhibitors (SSRIs), 110, 113

Serenity Prayer, 147

Serotonergic system, anxiety and, 52–53

Serotonin and norepinephrine reuptake inhibitors (SNRIs), 110, 113

Shelley, Mary, 170

Shell shock, 89

Shyness and Social Phobia, 87

Simple Phobia. *See* Specific Phobia (Simple Phobia)

Skin, responses to stress and anxiety of, 71

Skinner, B. F., 59

Sleep patterns and stress management, 150

Sleep-Related Problems (SRPs), 35

SNRIs. *See* Serotonin and norepinephrine reuptake inhibitors (SNRIs)

Social Anxiety Disorder. *See* Social Phobia (Social Anxiety Disorder)

Social Phobia (Social Anxiety Disorder), 6, 85, 86–89; attention training techniques and, 63; biological theories for, 51; characteristics of, 87;

comorbid conditions of, 88; diagnosis of, 89; men *vs.* women with, 86–87; physical symptoms of, 87–88; predictors of, 61; shyness and, 87; treatments for, 127–28

Social worker, 142, 144–45

Somatization Disorder, 158–60; diagnostic criteria for, 158–59; history of, 158; treatment for, 159–60

Somatoform Disorders, 151–68; Body Dysmorphic Disorder as, 165–67; Conversion Disorder as, 160–63; Factitious Disorders and, 152–55; Hypochondriasis as, 155–58; Malingering Disorders and, 152–55; overview of, 151–52; Pain Disorder as, 163–65; Somatization Disorder as, 158–60; Undifferentiated, 168

Specific Phobia (Simple Phobia), 6, 85–86; African Americans and, 40; common types of, 85; definition of, 85–86; lifetime prevalence of, 85; treatments for, 86, 128–29

Specific Social Disorder. *See* Social Phobia (Social Anxiety Disorder)

Split Personality, 176

SRPs. *See* Sleep-Related Problems (SRPs)

SSRIs. *See* Selective serotonin reuptake inhibitors (SSRIs)

Stevenson, Robert Lewis, 170

Strange Case of Dr. Jekyll and Mr. Hyde (Stevenson), 170

Stress management, 147–50; basic fundamentals of, 148; rules of, 148; strategies for, 149–50

Stressor, defined, 148

Substance abuse, anxiety-like symptoms of, 72

Substance-Induced Anxiety Disorder, 6

Suicide rate: for Alaskan Native young men, 45; for Native American young men, 45

Superstitious thinking, 9

Sybil, 170

Taijin kyôfu, 43

TCAs. *See* Tricyclic antidepressants (TCAs)

Teens, anxiety in, 32–36; comorbid conditions and, 35; diagnosing, 32–34; Sleep-Related Problems and, 35; treating, 35–36

Tetracyclics, 113

Theories of Anxiety Disorder, 49–67; biological, 49–54; integrating, 64–65; overview of, 49; patient vulnerability and, 65–67; psychological, 54–64

Thorndike, Edwin, 59

Threat, perceived *vs.* real, 2–3

Three Faces of Eve, The, 170, 178

Time management as stress management strategy, 149

Timothy's Law, 191

Tranquilizers, 111–12

Traumatic neurosis, 90

Treatments for Anxiety Disorders, 107–23; considerations in, 135–38; effects of, 145–47; elderly and, 137–38; Generalized Anxiety Disorder, 126–27; medical, 109–16; Mexican American youth and, 136–37; Obsessive-Compulsive Disorder, 130–33; overview of, 107–9; Panic Disorder, 125–26; Post-traumatic Stress Disorder, 133–35; psychological, 116–19; psychosocial approaches to, 119–23; Social Phobia (Social Anxiety Disorder), 127–28; Specific Phobia (Simple Phobia), 128–29

Tricyclic antidepressants (TCAs), 111, 114

Truth serum/drugs, 163

Undifferentiated Somatoform Disorder, 168

Vitamin B_{12} deficiency, anxiety-like symptoms of, 72

Von Munchausen, Baron, 153

White, Eve, 178

Women: anxiety and, 30–31; Post-traumatic Stress Disorder and, 91, 93–94; Specific Phobias and, 85

World Health Organization, 5

About the Author

RUDY NYDEGGER is a clinical psychologist and has a private practice and consulting firm. He is a professor of management and psychology at Union Graduate College and Union College and is chief of psychology as Ellis Hospital. He is a diplomate in clinical psychology through the American Board of Professional Psychology and is a fellow in the American Academy of Clinical Psychology. Nydegger was recently appointed to the board of the National Register of Health Service Providers in Psychology. He is married to Karen Nydegger and has four daughters, one son, and two grandsons.